Supporting Children and Families

of related interest

Improving Children's Services Networks
Lessons from Family Centres
Jane Tunstill, Jane Aldgate and Marilyn Hughes
ISBN 978 1 84310 461 2

Working with Parents of Young People
Research, Policy and Practice
Edited by Debi Roker and John Coleman
ISBN 978 1 84310 420 9

Costs and Outcomes in Children's Social Care
Messages from Research
Jennifer Beecham and Ian Sinclair
Foreword by Parmjit Dhanda MP
ISBN 978 1 84310 496 4

Child Protection, Domestic Violence and Parental Substance Misuse
Family Experiences and Effective Practice
Hedy Cleaver, Don Nicholson, Sukey Tarr and Deborah Cleaver
ISBN 978 1 84310 582 4
Quality Matters in Children's Services series

Handbook for Practice Learning in Social Work and Social Care
Knowledge and Theory
2nd edition
Edited by Joyce Lishman
ISBN 978 1 84310 186 4

The Post-Qualifying Handbook for Social Workers
Edited by Wade Tovey
ISBN 978 1 84310 428 5

Competence in Social Work Practice
A Practical Guide for Students and Professionals
2nd edition
Edited by Kieran O'Hagan
ISBN 978 1 84310 485 8

Getting Wise to Drugs
A Resource for Teaching Children about Drugs, Dangerous Substances and Other Risky Situations
David Emmett and Graeme Nice
ISBN 978 1 84310 507 7

Mental Health Interventions and Services for Vulnerable Children and Young People
Edited by Panos Vostanis
ISBN 978 1 84310 489 6

Understanding School Refusal
A Handbook for Professionals in Education, Health and Social Care
M.S. Thambirajah, Karen J. Grandison and Louise De-Hayes
ISBN 978 1 84310 567 1

Supporting Children and Families

Lessons from Sure Start for Evidence-Based Practice in Health, Social Care and Education

Edited by Justine Schneider, Mark Avis and Paul Leighton

Jessica Kingsley Publishers
London and Philadelphia

First published in 2007
by Jessica Kingsley Publishers
116 Pentonville Road
London N1 9JB, UK
and
400 Market Street, Suite 400
Philadelphia, PA 19106, USA

www.jkp.com

Library of Congress Cataloging in Publication Data
Supporting children and families : lessons from Sure Start for evidence-based practice in health, social care and education / edited by Justine Schneider, Mark Avis and Paul Leighton.
 p. cm.
 ISBN 978-1-84310-506-0 (pb : alk. paper) 1. Sure Start (Programme) 2. Children with social disabilities--Services for--Great Britain. 3. Day care centers--Great Britain. 4. Early childhood education--Great Britain. 5. Family services--Great Britain. 6. Medical care--Great Britain. I. Schneider, Justine. II. Avis, Mark. III. Leighton, Paul.
 HV751.A6S85 2007
 362.71--dc22

                                                                      2007032742

British Library Cataloguing in Publication Data
A CIP catalogue record for this book is available from the British Library

ISBN 978 1 84310 506 0

Printed and bound in Great Britain by
Athenaeum Press, Gateshead, Tyne and Wear

Note on changes to the structure of government departments in June 2007
In the course of writing this book two new government departments relating to this publication were set up by the Prime Minister on 28 June 2007:

- The Department for Children, Schools and Families (DCSF)
- The Department for Innovation, Universities and Skills (DIUS)

These new departments replaced the Department for Education and Skills (DfES), which is mentioned extensively in this book.

The Department for Children, Schools and Families (DCSF) is responsible for improving the focus on all aspects of policy affecting children and young people.

Contents

Part 5:   *Community Development*

List of Figures

List of Tables

Box

Chapter 1

Introduction: Sure Start in Context

Justine Schneider, Mark Avis and Paul Leighton

Sure Start was conceived as a means to promote the development and education of children (Eisenstadt 2002). Given impetus by the 2000 Comprehensive Spending Review, between 1999 and 2004, £1907 million (Department for Education and Skills (DfES) 2004) was allocated to 524 programmes in the most disadvantaged communities in England with a population of 400,000 pre-school children, a cost of about £4770 per capita. In November 2004, a new strategy for children was launched, with a new vision for Children's Centres, effectively marking a sea change in the nature of the Sure Start initiative. This book is the product of a national conference organised in Nottingham in June 2006 to bring together evaluators of Sure Start Local Programmes and to consolidate our findings from what had effectively been a massive social experiment.

Sure Start was set up with explicit outcome targets 'to achieve better outcomes for children, parents and communities by: increasing the availability of childcare for all children; improving health, education and emotional development for young children; supporting parents as parents and in their aspirations towards employment' (Kurtz 2003).

The key Sure Start aims of improving health, education and emotional development are clearly interlinked, since a child with emotional or health-related needs may not be able to take full advantage of educational opportunities, and both physical and emotional development are central aspects of education in young children. Sure Start, like many early years programmes, focused on the holistic needs of young children. Unlike any previous initiative, however, Sure Start programmes committed themselves to several fundamental principles: the involvement of parents in every aspect of the programme, coordination with existing local services to bring added value, cultural sensitivity and the avoidance of stigma. How local programmes achieved the aims of Sure Start by following these principles and what they discovered in doing so is the subject of this book.

Sure Start Local Programmes (SSLPs) were obliged to submit annual evaluation reports to the national coordinating centre. The National Evaluation of

Sure Start (NESS) website acts as a repository of at least 350 examples of these reports. In addition, on six-monthly returns throughout the duration of the agreement, between 2000 and 2004 when the Public Service Agreement (PSA) was revised, SSLPs had to produce reports on their progress towards the achievement of specific, quantified targets:

- *Social and emotional development*: a measured increase in the proportion of babies and young children aged 0–5 with normal levels of personal, social and emotional development for their age.

- *Health*: a percentage point reduction in the proportion of mothers who continue to smoke during pregnancy.

- *Ability to learn*: a percentage increase in the proportion of children having normal levels of communication, language and literacy, and an increase in the proportion of young children with satisfactory speech and language development at age two years.

- *Strengthening families*: a 12 per cent reduction in the proportion of young children (aged 0–4) living in households where no-one is working.

This requirement to report periodically tended to distract programme managers from the broader impact of their SSLPs and to drive the outputs of local evaluations. As programmes grew larger and more aspects fell under the evaluation spotlight, the reports became something of a treadmill, leaving little time for assimilation of the findings.

The national evaluation produced valuable syntheses of local reports on particular topics. These are also available on the NESS website, and include:

- speech and language services
- partnership working
- nutrition and breastfeeding support
- cost-effectiveness
- improving the employability of parents
- smoking cessation services
- black and minority ethnic families.

We do not seek to duplicate the synthesis reports, nor to summarise local evaluation reports here. Rather, this book takes major themes which emerged from the wider Sure Start experience and illustrates them from the perspectives of a small number of local evaluations. This collection is an attempt to take stock, to reflect on the Sure Start experience at greater length than time permitted during the operation of the first SSLPs. It brings together evidence from different SSLPs around child development and health, working in partnership, parental employment, supporting families, and community development. In this way, we hope to provide an overview of Sure Start that is more general than a single programme, yet more descriptive and nuanced than a synthesis can provide. This book helps to bridge the gap between the hundreds of local evaluation reports and the national evaluation reports.

There is a wealth of empirical evidence generated by Sure Start which should contribute to the advancement of knowledge in community development, early years studies, public health, education and other disciplines. The local evaluation reports alone contain material for dozens of PhD theses. This book demonstrates how the bridge between evidence and more general knowledge may be built. Current and future developments in services will be nourished and sustained by the Sure Start experience if we are able to draw evidence-based and defensible lessons from the vast amounts of data collected.

Many effective and creative projects within Sure Start programmes have not been fully described and documented. In some cases they are buried in evaluation reports and in others the results have taken longer to emerge. In addition to describing some innovative projects, we have tried here to draw more general inferences from the front line. At the end of each chapter the authors have highlighted three lessons for Children's Centres. These lessons are both tactical and strategic, and they are summarised in our concluding discussion.

It need hardly be pointed out that this represents an independent voice on Sure Start. Although the evaluations were centrally funded, they were commissioned by local programmes. Most of the evaluators enjoy the freedom of expression that goes with a university post. When the papers were presented in Nottingham in June 2006, most of the evaluations had been completed and the first five years of Sure Start funding had come to an end. The analyses presented here are therefore not constrained by considerations of local politics or by adherence to national policy.

As 'Sure Start Children's Centres' build on the foundations of Sure Start, this book offers a synthesis of some of the experiences which may be relevant. Of course, a new initiative will make its own mark, but previous work in a Sure Start setting has inevitably shaped the outlook of people who currently staff Children's Centres, as well as shaping the expectations of families. It is therefore vital to understand this experience and its many facets. The present book seeks to contribute to knowledge in this way.

References

Department for Education and Skills (DfES) (2004) Departmental Report. Cm 6202. Norwich: HMSO.

Eisenstadt, N. (2002) 'Sure Start: key principles and ethos.' Child: Care, Health and Development 28, 3–4.

Kurtz, Z. (2003) 'Outcomes for children's health and wellbeing.' Children and Society 17, 173–183.

Part 1

Health and Child Development

Chapter 2

Introduction to Health and Child Development

Mark Avis

From the outset, development of the Sure Start Programme was based on a recognition that the earliest years of a child's life were the most significant in their physical, social and emotional development. During the 1990s there had been mounting evidence of a cycle of interaction between the factors leading to social exclusion, such as poor educational attainment and reduced rates of participation in work, and poor health. The Independent Inquiry into Inequality in Health chaired by the government's then Chief Medical Officer, Sir Donald Acheson, reported that inequalities in health are of long standing and their determinants are deeply ingrained in our social structure (Acheson 1998). The underlying reasons for these inequalities in health were thought to start in the early years of a child's life and to persist across generations within families. Yet, at the same time, the predominant view of health services aimed at the under fours in the UK was that they were dislocated, uncoordinated and patchy, particularly so in areas of multiple disadvantage where children are especially vulnerable to environmental influences (Glass 1999).

Sure Start was to be an integrated response to these observed health inequalities; it was designed to be a community-based programme of intervention that could break the links between poor health and social exclusion. It was anticipated that a range of early interventions could lead to improvements in children's emotional and cognitive development, reduce the incidence of childhood ill health and accidents, and promote parents' confidence and self-sufficiency. In turn, these benefits would lead to improved education attainment and acquisition of work-related skills for both children and parents. Ultimately, over many years, these social benefits would have an impact on the Treasury through increased participation in the labour force and reduction in the costs of ill health and social exclusion, such as long-term disability, drug abuse, mental ill health and teenage pregnancy.

It is important to recognise that there was to be no 'national blueprint' for local interventions but that each local Sure Start Programme would, in responding to its local community, be based on some key principles. These were that interventions would be aimed at parents as well as children, that interventions and services should be delivered in a manner to avoid labelling and targeting of 'problem families', and that Sure Start Programmes would be multifaceted, attempting to integrate and add value to existing services in education, health, social care and leisure.

Although there was no blueprint for Sure Start interventions, each Sure Start Local Programme was required to offer core services and develop local targets that were informed by national targets as well as local needs and circumstances. The core offer for child and family health services included the provision of antenatal advice and support for parents, information and advice on breastfeeding, children's nutrition, prevention of infections and accidents in the under fives, identification of mothers at risk of postnatal depression, and smoking cessation services. These were linked to the development of national targets that reflected the available evidence on factors linked with inequalities in health. In particular, these included increasing the mean birthweight of babies, improving breastfeeding rates at one month and at three months, as well as decreasing the number of childhood accidents, reducing smoking rates amongst parents, and reducing the incidence of maternal mental ill health. In most cases conclusive evidence regarding the long-term impact of Sure Start interventions to address health inequalities will await larger-scale and longer-term studies. The local evaluations that we report in this chapter are largely concerned with what might be termed the process outputs of interventions, uptake of services, parental satisfaction and acceptability, and short-term outcomes in terms of breastfeeding rates and attendances by children under five at Accident and Emergency. Nonetheless, there is much to learn about how to make services attractive and engaging, and how to work with parents to enable them to believe that they can take actions that will have a positive impact on their own health and the health of their children.

The examples of local interventions contained in Part 1 of this book illustrate some of the ways in which Sure Start Local Programmes have addressed Sure Start health targets. One of the encouraging aspects of Sure Start has been the opportunity it gave to health professionals to think about new and innovative ways of integrating services. The Pampering Group described by Perry in Chapter 3 is a good example of an intervention that breaks new ground by bringing together expectant as well as new parents in an informal environment that was designed to lead to health and social benefits. It also illustrates a theme that recurs in many Sure Start interventions: an attempt to deliver services and advice in an informal, non-institutional manner that relies on making an intervention attractive to the people who are the intended beneficiaries. The Pampering Group was designed to address objectives that integrated health and social care benefits, such as improvement in breastfeeding rates, reduction in smoking during pregnancy, and improvements in parenting skills, all in the context of activities that were attractive and fun. This theme of making services more 'user friendly' is continued by Potter in Chapter 4: evaluating a Sure Start initiative to improve breastfeeding rates. Links between breastfeeding and improvements in childhood health are now well established. What is noticeable in Potter's account of a successful breastfeeding initiative is the emphasis that was placed on enhancing professionals' relationships with mothers and the active help of a peer support group. The value of supporting parents to deliver breastfeeding support is confirmed in the synthesis report on breastfeeding produced by the National Evaluation of Sure Start (NESS) (Latham *et al.* 2006). In this model, the focus of professional intervention shifts from dispensing individual advice to mothers to ways of incorporating and pooling the collective positive experiences of other parents.

Achieving a reduction in childhood accidents has been a long-term aim of several government initiatives. This goal was particularly relevant to Sure Start Local Programmes since it was thought that there is a link between social deprivation and the chances of a childhood accident (Department of Health 1999). Consequently many Sure Start Local Programmes actively pursued child injury prevention projects through the provision of home safety equipment, advice and education. However, it is not yet clear whether the provision of home safety equipment can be successful in reducing accidents in the home. In Chapter 5 Carman and colleagues describe the impact of a child injury prevention project based on a home consultation and provision of safety equipment coupled with a community-wide education and information programme. In exploring the impact of the programme the authors suggest that an effective community education campaign was central to its success. It is worth noting that the work on which this chapter is based has been recognised by the Audit Commission and Healthcare Commission (2007) as an example of good practice in their recent, jointly published report, *Better Safe than Sorry*.

In addition to allowing health professionals to innovate, Sure Start initiatives also provided an opportunity for health and early years staff to understand and recognise the need for specialist interventions for some families. The provision of training and integrated working with speech and language services and mental health provision within Sure Start Local Programmes has led to an 'added value' as a result of the increased knowledge and confidence that staff have gained in addressing such issues as language development or a mother's mental health problems. Potter and Hodgson's evaluation of a staff training course designed to improve the quality of language environment in pre-school settings was able to show that nursery nurses were more aware of opportunities and methods to enrich the communication environment (Chapter 6). The results of a synthesis of Sure Start local evaluations of speech and language initiatives published by NESS (Myers, Barnes and Kapoor 2005) confirm the importance of staff developing competence in issues around communication and having the ability to enrich interactions and communication environments.

Postnatal depression and maternal mental health problems remain stubbornly difficult to address because they are not well understood or widely discussed. It is not easy to explain the persistence of negative attitudes to people with mental health problems since the experience of having mental health problems is so widespread. Yet most health professionals find it difficult to talk about mental health issues, especially in the context of parenthood. The impact of parenthood on a mother's mental health is only just beginning to be recognised as a cause for concern. The experience of motherhood is not always as rewarding or fulfilling as expected, and many new mothers report feelings of social isolation, loss of confidence, and persistent tiredness and low mood. It is likely that many mothers who are experiencing low mood, and may be at risk of postnatal depression, would benefit from early identification of their problems and the timely provision of local help and support, both of which may have an impact on their mood as well as their parenting. Hall and Finnigan (Chapter 7) describe a Sure Start project to provide consultancy and training in maternal mental health to local family health services. Their chapter illustrates the difficulty in trying to evaluate a service that attempts to address the stigma associated with having a mental health problem, and the lack of confidence that many health professionals experience when having to address maternal mental health problems. However, the qualitative evidence they include suggests that a consultation service and education on the topic of maternal mental health can make an impact on professionals' confidence in addressing a difficult issue.

It should not be surprising that the health interventions evaluated in these chapters will also be central to the success of children's centres. The core offer for children's centres has to include antenatal advice and support, information and guidance on breastfeeding, hygiene, nutrition and safety, identification, care and support for those suffering from maternal depression, speech and language and other specialist support, and smoking cessation interventions. The examples provided in Part 1 of this book give some indications of good practice in these areas. They highlight the lessons that have been learnt in shifting the role of the professional from someone who dispenses advice and information to someone who mobilises community resources and support to promote breastfeeding, reduce accidents, and help people stop smoking. We have also learnt that professionals need to consider their own education as well as that of the rest of the community when tackling issues like maternal ill health and responsibility for home safety that people find difficult to talk about.

References

Acheson, D. (1998) *Independent Inquiry into Inequality in Health Report.* London: The Stationery Office.

Audit Commission and Healthcare Commission (2007) *Better Safe than Sorry: Preventing Unintentional Injury to Children.* London: Audit Commission.

Department of Health (1999) *Saving Lives: Our Healthier Nation.* London: HMSO.

Glass, N. (1999) 'Sure Start: the development of an early intervention programme for young children in the UK.' *Children and Society 13*, 257–264.

Latham, P., Kapoor, S., Myers, P. and Barnes, J. (2006) *Breastfeeding, Weaning and Healthy Eating: A Synthesis of Sure Start Local Programme Evaluation Findings.* London: Birkbeck College (University of London), National Evaluation of Sure Start (NESS).

Myers, P., Barnes, J. and Kapoor, S. (2005) *Speech and Language Services in Sure Start Local Programmes. Findings from Local Evaluations.* London: Birkbeck College (University of London), National Evaluation of Sure Start (NESS).

Chapter 3

Evaluation of a Pampering Group

Catherine Perry

The Pampering Group at the Sure Start Widnes Trailblazer Programme provides health and beauty treatments for parents-to-be and new parents, as well as an opportunity for informal advice and support from other parents and professionals about childbirth and parenting a young child. It is held on a weekly basis and is organised by a multidisciplinary team, including a family support worker, midwife, health visitor, massage and beauty therapist, community food coordinator and maternity care assistant. The activities are intended to provide physical relaxation, emotional support, pragmatic advice and an opportunity for local parents to get to know each other.

The whole approach is based on evidence of the health risks of certain behaviours, such as the effects of smoking during pregnancy on birth weight (Spencer 2004), and the positive health outcomes of other behaviours, such as breastfeeding (Kramer and Kakuma 2002). In addition, providing practical and social support for parents living in disadvantaged conditions is likely to help improve outcomes for children (Department of Health 2004), while reducing isolation for parents is important in increasing self-esteem and can improve parenting (Grimshaw and McGuire 1998).

This chapter presents some of the findings from a small-scale, qualitative, exploratory study designed to investigate the extent to which the Pampering Group had fulfilled its aim and objectives. It reflects on what appeared to work and why, and considers how such service provision could be integrated with current specifications for Children's Centres.

The study

The study utilised three qualitative data collection methods (observation, semistructured interviews and a focus group) to describe the service and to record perceptions about its benefits and limitations, according to both users and providers. A grounded theory approach was used in the research (Glaser and Strauss 1967), allowing data collection to be refined in the light of data gathered.

A researcher observed the Pampering Group on two occasions. Notes were taken during the observation sessions using an observation framework. The data from observation sessions were used to provide a 'thick description' of the functioning of the Pampering Group on the occasions when the researcher was present. This allowed the interview and focus group data to be interpreted in context, and also allows the transferability of the findings to other settings to be assessed.

Semistructured interviews were conducted with parents who had attended the Pampering Group on more than one occasion (six individuals, one of whom was the mother of twins), and with professionals who referred parents to the group but did not have any further involvement with it (two midwives). A focus group was carried out with the professionals involved in providing the Pampering Group. Three professionals (one midwife and two family support workers) took part in the focus group and one involved professional (a health visitor) was interviewed on her own, as she was unable to attend at the time of the focus group. With each participant's permission, the interviews and focus group were tape-recorded. The tapes were then transcribed verbatim. The interview and focus group data were combined and the transcripts subjected to thematic analysis. These findings were used to draw conclusions about the Pampering Group in relation to its aim and objectives and its contribution to the work of the Sure Start Local Programme.

Permission to carry out the study was sought from Cheshire Local Research Ethics Committee and gained in July 2004.

Findings from the study

Those involved in the Pampering Group were, on the whole, extremely enthusiastic about it and keen to see it developed. By using the objectives of the Pampering Group as a framework for the findings that follow, what becomes evident is where the Pampering Group has achieved success and what can be learnt from the experience to inform future service development.

Preparation for childbirth

The Pampering Group aimed to help parents to feel emotionally and practically prepared for childbirth. However, although some women had attended the group whilst pregnant and perceived it to be a beneficial experience, very few pregnant women had attended in total, and those who had did not tend to return. One reason for non-attendance suggested by study interviewees was that often women did not learn about the group antenatally. In Widnes, midwives are required to tell women about Sure Start services when they book in for maternity care. This is a time when a lot of information is given, and some professionals felt that information about activities such as the Pampering Group would not be taken on board by women. None of the women interviewed recalled hearing about the Pampering Group from a midwife, indicating either that they had failed to retain the information, or that the midwives were not passing the information on. There was also evidence in the interviews with professionals of a lack of clarity about the Pampering Group among those potentially referring women. This suggests that opportunities for publicising the group effectively were lost.

Second, it was suggested that women felt 'left out' if they did not have a baby at the Pampering Group. There was a perception that, although all women were welcomed into the group by the professionals and the other women, attention was focused on the mothers of young babies. One professional described how a pregnant woman told her that she had been to the Pampering Group but thought she was in the wrong place because everybody had a baby and was talking about them: the babies were often the catalyst for conversations. Indeed, in one of the observation sessions, a pregnant woman was observed to have little interaction with other mothers, although she did interact with professionals. Therefore, it may be that the group was not a comfortable environment for pregnant women.

Support for parents

There were a number of ways in which the Pampering Group aimed to support parents: by identifying those women at risk of postnatal depression and providing treatment if necessary; by fostering self-care and infant care; by increasing parents' self-confidence; and through increasing parents' self-efficacy and social cohesion. Each of these is explored below.

POSTNATAL DEPRESSION

One of the objectives of the group was to identify those at risk of postnatal depression and to provide treatment if necessary. Because of the way in which the group was conducted, with a great deal of informal contact between women attending and staff, there were likely to be ample opportunities for health professionals to 'pick up' any indications of postnatal depression. There was evidence in the findings of this study that both professionals and mothers considered the Pampering Group to be helpful in combating mild levels of depression. Professionals gave examples of women whom they considered had been helped in this way, and women themselves spoke of their own experiences of depression and how the Pampering Group had helped them. Two women in particular, who had been referred by health visitors because of worries about depression, credited the Pampering Group with helping them to enjoy parenting and overcome the challenges they faced.

The mechanism by which this was achieved appeared to be twofold. First, social support was generated by the Pampering Group. Women met others in similar situations and were able to help and encourage each other. The peer support offered was evidenced both in the observation sessions and the interviews. One woman commented:

> Then once I got out and I got to the Pampering Group and you see lots of other mums who are having a similar experience then that helped. But when I was isolated and not going anywhere and not doing anything, I thought it was only happening to me.

In addition, many of the women at the group had formed friendships and met up outside the group. One woman commented that since she had her baby and joined the Pampering Group, her social life had 'gone through the roof', an experience that would not usually be associated with new motherhood!

Women also commented on the perceived 'social benefit' that their babies derived from the Pampering Group. Babies were often talked to and played with by adults other than their parent at the group, and although too young to have much sustained interaction with other babies, it was believed that the babies benefited from each others' company.

Second, the treatments offered were perceived to be important as they focused on the mother and gave her some individual attention, at a time when almost all attention would be centred on the newborn baby. One woman commented: 'For me it is like an added bonus, it is nice. That is the only "me" time I get'.

FOSTERING SELF-CARE AND INFANT CARE

At the Pampering Group, most health education and promotion activity took place in an informal way between the women themselves and between the professionals present and the women: this appeared to be a successful approach. For example, one mother talked about how her experience had helped another woman, struggling with breastfeeding, to breastfeed twins successfully. Another example of informal health promotion around self and infant care was the food available at the Pampering Group sessions. Each week, a selection of healthy food was available for the women attending the group, and for their babies, if appropriate. It was evident in the observation sessions that the food was a central feature of the group. Both mothers and babies were observed trying food that they had not eaten before. Many of the interactions and discussions between the parents centred on food and the feeding of children. By having healthy food available, discussion about healthy eating for adults and children was encouraged.

The staff perceived that more could be done in terms of formal health promotion in the Pampering Group, and plans for short talks about self and infant care to become a feature of the group were suggested. However, it would seem important that this does not stifle more informal channels of information as the informality was valued by the women.

The treatments were a very obvious way in which self-care was encouraged and enabled at the Pampering Group. They gave a clear message about the legitimacy of self-care, and comments were made about how helpful and enjoyable they could be. It was evident, however, that all the participating professionals and the users of the group perceived the treatments, although important, to be secondary to the social aspect of the group. One woman commented: 'No one is ever bothered if they don't get one [treatment] because you have still had a good laugh and a chat and a drink and watched your babies playing and stuff'.

INCREASING PARENTS' CONFIDENCE

The women who were interviewed for this study were relatively confident about their parenting ability. They were, in general, from large, close families or were experienced parents already. However, most commented that they had seen the group help other, younger or less experienced mothers, and they perceived that the group was very beneficial in educating people about parenting and improving their confidence. In addition, even experienced mothers, or those who were professionally experienced with children, commented that the group had helped to give them confidence in themselves as mothers. One woman commented: 'It doesn't matter how much experience you have got looking after other people's babies. It didn't prepare me for looking after my own and I think it has helped in that respect greatly'.

The women all reported that the sharing of knowledge between parents and between parents and health professionals in the group had the capacity to improve their confidence and competence. In particular, women articulated that sometimes, if they were worried about what they regarded as a trivial matter, they were able to bring it up during the Pampering Group, although they would probably not have made a specific telephone call or seen a health visitor to ask for advice. One woman commented:

> Sometimes you feel stupid getting on the phone to the health visitor…[if you have] just changed the consistency of her food a little tiny bit and you feel stupid. But when you are just talking then, people say, "Oh, yes". So then you got confidence in your own thoughts then.

INCREASING SELF-EFFICACY AND SOCIAL COHESION

The Pampering Group aimed to increase the self-efficacy of parents and enable them to engage in the local community. Striking evidence of the success of the Pampering Group in increasing self-efficacy was provided by a follow-on group set up by parents who formerly attended the Pampering Group. This group was organised entirely by parents whose children had outgrown the Pampering Group and was run by parent volunteers. During the interviews a great deal of pride in this achievement was voiced, as well as enthusiasm for the new group. In addition to this, evidence of widening circles of friends, and peer support outside the Pampering Group, was contained in the interview data. Women reported visiting each other at home regularly, going for nights out and staying in touch as their children grew older. It is possible that, as the parents get to know each other, a 'snowball' effect of friendships develops as each woman introduces another into a wider social network.

Discussion

The findings presented here indicate that parents and professionals involved with the Pampering Group perceived it to be largely successful, and indicate some of the ways in which this was so. Although there is little empirical evidence in the research literature specifically about pampering groups, there are a number of indications that a group such as this one should be able to provide valuable support to parents and parents-to-be.

North (undated) argues that antenatal care that focuses only on medical aspects of pregnancy and birth does not meet the needs of parents, and that non-traditional care that includes group discussion and plentiful involvement of midwives can reduce infant mortality and increase birth weight. In addition, the literature indicates that supplementary contact with a health visitor postnatally can be effective in preventing depression (Cooper *et al.* 2003; Murray, Woolgar and Cooper 2004). Postnatal care that facilitates peer support can also help to promote healthy behaviours (North undated). There is evidence that the use of massage and relaxation techniques can reduce stress (Field 2000; Risberg *et al.* 2004), and providing such treatments to pregnant women and the mothers of young babies is likely to be useful in terms of their health, self-esteem and well-being. Health promoting behaviour has been demonstrated to be inextricably linked to high self-esteem, feeling valued and feeling part of a community (D'Souza and Garcia 2004; Vimpani 2000). The Pampering Group provided an opportunity for women to learn about self-care and infant care, while helping to foster the improvements in self-esteem and inclusion in the community that help in their successful application. Finally, a mini service evaluation of the Pampering Group at another Sure Start Local Programme concluded that the Pampering Group was an innovative approach to providing emotional and social support and health advice to antenatal and postnatal women, and had an important role in introducing pregnant women to each other and to other Sure Start services (Rouse, Barrow and Thurston 2004). The group's structure and format was thus evidence-based, as it is known that providing supportive groups and pragmatic help in order to reduce social isolation helps young families to foster good mental and physical health (Grimshaw and McGuire 1998; North undated).

Children's Centres will be charged with providing, amongst other services, antenatal and postnatal services, information on parenting, drop-in groups, and opportunities for parents to access parenting support and education

(Department for Education and Skills 2005). Therefore, it is clear that the Pampering Group model is one which could be taken forward and integrated into the Children's Centre agenda. As guidance for Children's Centres indicates that the views of parents should be taken into account in the planning of services (Department for Education and Skills 2005), findings from studies such as this can be utilised to aid decision-making about the configuration of services. Four issues highlighted in this evaluation would seem to be particularly pertinent.

The nature of the support offered

There was evidence in this study that the Pampering Group was successful in supporting women postnatally, both personally and as mothers, in caring for their babies. The nature of the support offered was holistic, informal and 'indirect', in that women attended the group not to hear a presentation about a particular aspect of parenting, but to be with and talk to other women in a similar situation, and to health and social care professionals. Some professional interviewees were concerned that there should be more formal health promotion sessions at the Pampering Group, but it would seem important that this does not stifle the informal channels of information which were valued by the women. This informality was non-threatening, encouraged a naturalistic setting and was dynamic, and there was thus an indirect pathway to outcomes. Sure Start Local Programmes have provided a 'test bed' for imaginative strategies for facilitating access (Garbers *et al.* 2006), and this indirect approach is one of them. The Pampering Group facilitated easy access to professionals and other parents so that an individual seeking advice could do so informally and unobtrusively. One of the premises on which the Children's Centre agenda will be carried forward is that seeking advice and help is the action of a responsible parent (Garbers *et al.* 2006), and the Pampering Group was enabling parents to achieve just this.

Targeting potential audiences

The Pampering Group was successful in attracting postnatal women, but did not have the same success in attracting antenatal women although, potentially, the diverse needs of pregnant women could be successfully met by the multi-faceted approach of the Pampering Group. In addition, groups who have been traditionally classed as 'hard-to-reach', such as younger women or fathers, were not accessing the service. It may be that the original target audience for the group – all parents and parents-to-be – is a group just too diverse to be attracted to, and supported by, one service. Services for parents and families need to be designed in a user-friendly way (Garbers *et al.* 2006), and if users are very diverse this might be difficult. The model of holistic, informal and indirect support offered at the Pampering Group may be a model that would work well if targeted at particular, more discrete, groups of parents: for example, antenatal women or young mothers. Young mothers, in particular, tend not to access traditional antenatal services (Health Development Agency 2001), but if there were a Pampering Group directed specifically at them, the accessible, non-threatening and informal atmosphere might be an opportunity to provide a way in for teenage parents to access support and advice from health professionals.

The issue of fathers is also worthy of comment. The Pampering Group was aimed at all parents, but no fathers attended. This may have been for numerous reasons, including that the group ran during the day or that the idea of 'pampering' was off-putting. However, if fathers had attended, this might have altered the dynamics of the group and detracted from the way in which the women were able to interact with and support each other. This is another example of how the target group – all parents and parents-to-be – may have been too diverse.

Publicising services

Publicising services has been described as a 'key building block in the access system' (Garbers *et al.* 2006, p.290). This study underlines the importance of adequate and timely publicity about the Pampering Group in relation to antenatal women. The services need to be publicised at a time and in a place where they are most likely to be seen and heard by their target audience. In addition, it is vital that information is regularly updated so that potential service users receive accurate details about services from which they might benefit.

Multidisciplinary team working

Delivering Children's Centre services requires a range of agencies and organisations to work together (Department for Education and Skills 2005). The Pampering Group was delivered by a multidisciplinary team and is an example of successful cross-boundary working, involving, as it did, a variety of professionals from health and social care and beyond. However, this way of working did raise some issues. For example, there was some evidence in the interviews of a lack of clarity about the Pampering Group among those potentially referring women in, indicating a need for these professionals to increase their knowledge base. This may reflect one of the issues that can arise with multidisciplinary working, in that midwives were directing women to a service with which they were not directly involved, and highlights the need for good communication between the different professional groups involved in a multidisciplinary project.

Conclusion and implications

The Pampering Group's activities were intended to give physical relaxation, emotional support, pragmatic advice and an opportunity for local parents to get to know and support each other. There is evidence in this study to suggest that the group achieved these objectives, particularly in relation to postnatal women. In the move to Children's Centres, these findings could help to inform service development, in particular the four points discussed above:

- the importance of thinking about the nature of support offered – in terms of issues such as formal/informal and direct/indirect support
- the targeting of potential audiences
- the importance of adequate and timely publicity
- the importance of communication in multidisciplinary team working.

Acknowledgements

Thanks go to the parents who participated in this research, and to the Pampering Group staff and other professionals who were interviewed. Thanks are also due to Denise Alexander for carrying out fieldwork. The evaluation was commissioned by Sure Start Widnes Trailblazer Local Programme and funded by Halton Borough Council (the accountable body).

References

Cooper, P.J., Murray, L., Wilson, A. and Romaniuk, H. (2003) 'Controlled trial of the short- and long-term effect of psychological treatment of post-partum depression.' *British Journal of Psychiatry 182*, 5, 412–419.

Department for Education and Skills (2005) *Sure Start Children's Centres: Practice Guidance.* London: DfES.

Department of Health (2004) *National Service Framework for Children, Young People and Maternity Services: Core Standards.* www.dh.gov.uk/assetRoot/04/09/05/66/04090566.pdf, accessed on 4 February 2005.

D'Souza, L. and Garcia, J. (2004) 'Improving services for disadvantaged childbearing women.' *Child: Care, Health and Development 30*, 6, 599–611.

Field, T. (2000) *Touch Therapy.* Edinburgh: Churchill Livingstone.

Garbers, C., Tunstill, J., Allnock, D. and Akhurst, S. (2006) 'Facilitating access to services for children and families: lessons from Sure Start Local Programmes.' *Child and Family Social Work 11*, 4, 287–296.

Glaser, B.G. and Strauss, A.L. (1967) *The Discovery of Grounded Theory: Strategies for Qualitative Research.* New York, NY: Aldine.

Grimshaw, R. and McGuire, C. (1998) *Evaluating Parenting Programmes.* www.jrf.org.uk/knowledge/findings/socialpolicy/SPR978.asp, accessed on 25 April 2005.

Health Development Agency (2001) *Teenage Pregnancy: an Update on Key Characteristics of Effective Interventions.* www.dfes.gov.uk/teenagepregnancy/dsp_showDoc.cfm?FileName=HDA%20review%2Epdf, accessed on 15 May 2005.

Kramer, M.S. and Kakuma, R. (2002). *The Optimum Duration of Exclusive Breastfeeding: a Systematic Review.* Geneva: WHO Publications.

Murray, L., Woolgar, M. and Cooper, P. (2004) 'Detection and treatments of postpartum depression.' *Community Practitioner 77*, 1, 13–17.

North, J. (undated) *Support from the Start. Lessons from International Early Years Policy.* London: Maternity Alliance.

Risberg, T., Kolstad, A., Bremnes, Y., Holte, H., Wist, E.A., Mella, O., Klepp, O., Wilsgaard, T. and Cassileth, B.R. (2004) 'Knowledge of and attitudes toward complementary and alternative therapies: a national multicentre study of oncology professionals in Norway.' *European Journal of Cancer Care 40,* 4, 529–535.

Rouse, J., Barrow, M. and Thurston, M. (2004) *Service Evaluation of the Sure Start Pampering Group.* Chester: Centre for Public Health Research, University College Chester.

Spencer, N. (2004) 'Accounting for the social disparity in birth weight: results from an intergenerational cohort.' *Journal of Epidemiology and Community Health 58,* 5, 418–419.

Vimpani, G. (2000). 'Child development and the civil society: does social capital matter?' *Journal of Developmental and Behavioural Paediatrics 21,* 1, 44–47.

Chapter 4

Increasing Breastfeeding Rates: Issues and Approaches

Carol Potter

Improving nutrition was identified early on as a major target area for Sure Start Local Programmes. Since it is known that breast milk provides the best nutritional start for health (Kohner 1997), programmes were charged with improving service delivery in the area of breastfeeding. A directive from the Department for Education and Skills (DfES) mandated that: 'All local programmes should give guidance on breastfeeding, hygiene and safety' (Department for Education and Skills 2002).

Known benefits of breastfeeding for children include a significantly reduced risk of infection (particularly gastrointestinal), as well as significant advantages in terms of cognitive function in both low weight and healthy full-term infants. For mothers, long-term health benefits include a reduced risk of breast cancer, some forms of ovarian cancer and osteoporosis (Villalpando and Hamosh 1998; Yngve and Sjostrom 2001). In addition, breast milk is known to reduce childhood obesity (Armstrong and Reilly 2002) as well as exerting a protective effect on the attainment of gross motor milestones (Sacker, Quigley and Kelly 2006). The interaction between mother and baby also helps to promote psychosocial adjustment (Fergusson and Woodward 1999).

Findings from UK infant feeding surveys, carried out every five years, indicate that there has been a steady increase in breastfeeding at birth in the UK, rising from 66 per cent in 1995 (Office of Population Censuses and Surveys (OPCS) 1995) to 77 per cent in 2005 (Bolling 2006). There are, however, significant variations in breastfeeding rates according to social class, age and area of the country. In 2005, 88 per cent of women from managerial and professional backgrounds breastfed initially, whilst only 65 per cent from manual labour backgrounds did so. In other words, babies from areas of disadvantage are much less likely to be breastfed than others. This was the situation which Sure Start Local Programmes aimed to change by increasing breastfeeding rates within their catchment areas.

A National Evaluation of Sure Start (NESS) synthesis report reviewed findings from 58 Sure Start Local Programme evaluation reports in the area of breastfeeding and found that there had been 'some evidence of an increase in the "initiation and duration" of breastfeeding rates measured over specific time scales' (Latham *et al.* 2006, p.3). NESS concluded that the range of strategies in use across programmes fell into three main categories, namely:

1. improving access to breastfeeding support for mothers in hospital
2. introducing peer support approaches
3. improving existing services and multidisciplinary working.

This chapter explores how one Sure Start programme in the north of England doubled its breastfeeding initiation rates from an extremely low baseline, within a two-year period, and has maintained this progress over time.

Methodology

Sure Start Felgate was one of a number of Sure Start programmes in the north of England which formed a consortium for the purposes of local evaluation. Having successfully tendered for the contract, Durham University began its work with the consortium in 2001. The day-to-day operation of the research was managed by a multidisciplinary research team within the then Centre for Applied Social Studies, whilst the strategic direction of the evaluation was managed by a steering group consisting of local programme managers and the University's research team.

Research questions for the study under discussion were:

- What are the perceived barriers to breastfeeding in the Sure Start Felgate area?
- What have been the rates of breastfeeding at birth and four weeks since the programme became operational in 2001?
- What factors have influenced breastfeeding rates during this period?
- What are mothers' views of professional support for breastfeeding in their local area?

Data discussed in this chapter are drawn from:

- Sure Start Felgate's database
- semistructured interviews with seven members of Sure Start staff: two midwives, the former health visitor coordinator, librarian, administrator, family support worker coordinator and two early years family support workers
- telephone interviews with six breastfeeding mothers.

Informed consent was obtained from all participants in the normal way: that is to say, participants were informed of the purpose of the evaluation and given guarantees of anonymity and confidentiality. Approval for a range of Sure Start local evaluation projects being undertaken by Durham University was gained from a Local Research Ethics Committee in 2003.

A purposive sample of Sure Start staff was interviewed (Robson 2002) (i.e. those who were thought to have important information relevant to the evaluation). A convenience sample of mothers was interviewed (Robson 2002) (i.e. mothers who were willing to take part in the evaluation). Their views, therefore, cannot be said to be representative of what other breastfeeding mothers may have thought. For the purposes of this study, they are intended to be of illustrative value only.

With regard to database information provided in the study, Sure Start Felgate midwives routinely collect information on feeding choice at birth and at four weeks, when health visitors take on the supporting clinical role. This information is regularly entered on the programme's database by Sure Start administrators, thereby ensuring an accurate picture of feeding choices within the area at any given time.

Findings
Barriers to breastfeeding

Sure Start Felgate health professionals reported that there were many complex cultural, personal and financial barriers to breastfeeding locally. One midwife commented: 'It's not just a matter of changing feeding practices, it's a matter of changing culture, which is a huge challenge'. Another health professional also noted that the culture of breastfeeding which existed in the area years ago had been lost:

> For the generation of local women now in their seventies, breastfeeding had been the norm and there was great skill and knowledge in the area. Mothers now have mostly bottle-fed, so this is the normal choice around here – there's been very little cultural support for breastfeeding for a lot of years.

The lack of a culture of breastfeeding, coupled with low incidence, has meant that few women in the area will have seen others breastfeeding which, in itself, is known to affect women's feeding choices. In fact, some of the mothers we spoke to in the Felgate area gave lack of contact with breastfeeding women as a reason for not having breastfed older children. One mother reported: 'I was terrified about doing it – no-one in our family had ever breastfed'. Another stated: 'None of my friends had [breastfed]...I didn't know anyone who had'.

Another perceived barrier to breastfeeding related to media images. Sure Start Felgate midwives thought that many first-time mothers appeared to have absorbed some unrealistic expectations of what having a baby and breastfeeding might be like from the media: 'The media is always showing pictures of perfect babies who eat and sleep when bottle-fed and although this picture is far from the reality, it's often very hard to persuade many women of this'. Such a perception fits well with research findings on how feeding methods are portrayed in the media. Henderson, Kitzinger and Green (2000) explored how breastfeeding and bottlefeeding were presented in a range of newspapers and television programmes during one month in 1999. They found that the two feeding methods were presented very differently, with bottlefeeding being portrayed more often as the feeding choice associated with fewer problems.

It is clear that the challenge involved in improving breastfeeding rates in the Felgate area was a significant one, a statement supported by breastfeeding rates reported during the first year of Sure Start Felgate's operation.

Breastfeeding rates

The proportion of women breastfeeding at birth in the Felgate area stood at only 25 per cent in 2001, compared with 57 per cent of mothers from social class 5 across the UK as a whole. That is to say, in the Sure Start Felgate catchment area, breastfeeding rates at birth stood at less than half the national average of women from similar socioeconomic backgrounds (Hamlyn *et al.* 2000). During the five years since 2001, Sure Start Felgate breastfeeding rates have increased significantly as shown below.

Table 4.1 Sure Start Felgate breastfeeding rates: 2001–2005

Year	Birth	4 weeks
2001	25%	9%
2002	38%	17%
2003	48%	34%
2004	44%	24%
2005	52%	23%

The rates also show a steady increase over time, from a very low baseline in the programme's first year. The increases appear to be due to three interrelated factors: the programme-wide implementation of the UNICEF Baby Friendly Initiative (BFI), an enhanced model of service delivery, and the setting up of two local groups where breastfeeding women could offer each other informal support, at the same time as influencing other mothers who were not currently breastfeeding.

The UNICEF Baby Friendly Initiative

A key strategy adopted by Sure Start Felgate to increase breastfeeding rates in the area was the implementation of the UNICEF Baby Friendly Initiative. The approach was first introduced into the programme in 2001 by the programme's then health visitor coordinator who was crucial in leading it within the programme. The process was also fully supported by Sure Start Felgate's then programme manager.

The BFI is a worldwide programme, developed by UNICEF and the World Health Organisation, which works with health services to improve practice in the area of breastfeeding. Specifically, it seeks to promote practice which ensures informed choice in the area of infant feeding, as well as high quality support for breastfeeding:

> The Baby Friendly Initiative works with the healthcare system to ensure a high standard of care for pregnant women and breastfeeding mothers and babies. We provide support for healthcare facilities who are seeking to implement best practice approaches. (UNICEF Baby Friendly 2001a)

The BFI was introduced into UK maternity services in 1993, by UNICEF UK Baby Friendly and the Department of Health, and in 1998 was extended to include community-based services. To achieve the prestigious Baby Friendly accreditation, services need to submit themselves to a rigorously monitored process which involves demonstrating compliance with a number of evidence-based standards: ten for hospitals and seven for community settings such as Sure Start Local Programmes. In community settings, providers should:

1. have a written breastfeeding policy that is routinely communicated to all healthcare staff

2. train all staff involved in the care of mothers and babies in the skills necessary to implement the policy

3. inform all pregnant women about the benefits and management of breastfeeding

4. support mothers to initiate and maintain breastfeeding

5. encourage exclusive and continued breastfeeding, with appropriately timed introduction of complementary foods

6. provide a welcoming atmosphere for breastfeeding families

7. promote cooperation between healthcare staff, breastfeeding support groups and the local community. (UNICEF Baby Friendly 2001b)

The full accreditation process consists of a number of steps, beginning with a register of intent to work towards Baby Friendly status which is followed by an action planning visit. A certificate of commitment is then awarded to signify that a provider has a breastfeeding policy in place, a plan through which to achieve Baby Friendly accreditation, and the commitment to implement the plan within two years. When a service believes that it has met all of the standards, UNICEF conducts the initial accreditation assessment, and often a follow-up visit, to ensure that any issues identified during the assessment have been addressed. A reassessment takes place 24 months after a healthcare facility is accredited as Baby Friendly and at regular intervals thereafter.

In 2006, 45 hospitals within the UK had gained Baby Friendly accredited status, as well as seven community settings, including Sure Start Felgate, which was one of the first Sure Start Local Programmes to achieve accreditation in November 2002. The programme succeeded in maintaining its Baby Friendly status at the point this chapter was written.

Impact of Baby Friendly training

An integral part of adopting the BFI is that key staff should undertake UNICEF training on breastfeeding. Midwives and health visitors attend a three-day course in breastfeeding management, whilst other staff who work in supporting roles, such as nursery nurses and healthcare assistants, attend a two-day course on helping mothers to breastfeed. Health professionals in Sure Start Felgate discussed the impact of the Baby Friendly training on their practice. One midwife stated: 'The course opened my eyes. I had been a midwife for 20 years and I learnt a lot I hadn't known before. I hadn't gone fully into the mechanics of positioning'. Staff also learnt much more than they had known about the benefits of breastfeeding, which clinical staff working within a Baby Friendly accredited programme are required to relay to pregnant women throughout their pregnancy, so that they can make much more of an informed choice.

An informed choice

Implementing BFI guidelines has required health professionals in Sure Start Felgate to make significant alterations to the way in which they approach discussing infant feeding choices with pregnant women. A key principle is that all women, regardless of the feeding decision they may already have made, are informed of the benefits of breastfeeding and how it can be achieved. Therefore, on first meeting pregnant women in Sure Start Felgate, midwives do not ask how women are going to feed their babies. Instead they say, 'I'd like to tell you about breastfeeding', conveying the impression that this is the normal way of feeding babies. One health visitor said: 'It's very rare that a woman will refuse to listen to the information and many are not aware of all of the issues when they do hear the facts about breastfeeding'.

According to Sure Start midwives, many women in their local area appear to believe the marketing information relating to the benefits of 'scientifically formulated' bottle milk. Midwives are required by Baby Friendly guidelines to provide information about the chemicals which are added to formula milk. Women are also reminded of the practical and financial benefits of breastfeeding, which include savings of over £400 and no need to sterilise feeding bottles.

Over the course of the pregnancy, Sure Start midwives present information relating to breastfeeding from a number of perspectives. For example, they talk about the natural animal instinct to feed their young, as well as the importance of skin-to-skin contact which calms babies, supports bonding and reduces temperature. Staff commented that even if women do not go on to breastfeed, many take on board information about the importance of skin-to-skin contact. Staff try to convey to women that it is not an 'all or nothing decision': women could 'give it a go' without committing themselves. This strategy has the effect of reducing the pressure on women to make a firm decision in favour of bottlefeeding. Overall, midwives take a gradual approach, giving women a little more information about the benefits of breastfeeding at each visit, to try to 'keep the momentum going'.

Sure Start health professionals agreed that the Baby Friendly compulsory information-giving approach was successful. One health visitor said: 'Women do change their mind about how they are going to feed their babies when they have all of the information'. Another stated:

> The piece of information which will make the difference in terms of decision-making varies between women. For some, it is the idea that they will not have to get out of bed to feed their baby, whereas for others it is the stated health benefits.

Some of the mothers we spoke to confirmed the effectiveness of the ongoing Baby Friendly approach to giving information. One mother told us how she had changed her mind about her feeding choice because of the information she received from the midwife, having previously 'already got the bottles in'. Another woman told us that it was the information on benefits to the immune system which affected her decision: 'A few months before I had the baby, the midwife told me that [in situations like mine], the baby's immune system could be affected – breast milk would give him his own protection – that's what did it'.

An integrated programme-wide approach

In Sure Start Felgate, all 26 staff attended Baby Friendly training to ensure a programme-wide approach, in which each member of staff could contribute to the promotion and maintenance of breastfeeding from within their own particular role. For example, following the course, the programme's librarian ensured that there were a number of practical books on breastfeeding available for women to borrow and to refer to in all programme venues. In addition, the librarian reported that what she had learnt on the UNICEF training enabled her to feel more confident when the subject of breastfeeding arose in informal conversations:

> When you make relationships with parents, you don't know what will come up in conversation – you need to know something about breastfeeding – so that you can be reassuring – and be able to direct women to the right person within the programme for advice.

Administrators are often the first point of call when women contact the programme or enter the Sure Start building. Having a non-clinical role, these staff cannot give advice on breastfeeding but are able to invite women to breastfeed on the premises and signpost them to those clinical staff within the programme who can do so. Queries from women regarding breastfeeding are given priority, and administrators will quickly contact relevant staff, wherever they are, so that advice will be forthcoming as quickly as possible. One mother commented on the speed of the programme's response to her request for help with breastfeeding: 'I phoned the programme office and the midwife was here within ten minutes – I couldn't believe it'.

Early years family support workers are another key group in providing ongoing support for breastfeeding mothers. Following their UNICEF training, they have been able to deliver informed advice on the benefits of breastfeeding, as well as on positioning and attachment to the breast, in the variety of contexts in which they work. For example, they are able to talk with women informally in play sessions, clinics and during family support visits. One early years family support worker commented: 'If we're working in one of the venues, we can sit and have a chat and ask how they're getting on with positioning…we can go through some advice or signpost the women to the relevant person in the programme'. In this way, breastfeeding women in the programme area can receive help and advice from a number of staff, in a range of contexts, not only from midwives during clinic appointments or home visits.

A community-wide approach

Baby Friendly standards for community settings require service providers to promote breastfeeding within the local community. In order to address the issue of women being extremely reluctant to breastfeed in public, Sure Start staff have regularly canvassed local shops in the town centre to lobby for acceptance of breastfeeding. This strategy was relatively successful with most shops agreeing to put breastfeeding friendly posters in their windows whilst, in some places, specific breastfeeding areas were established as a result of programme lobbying.

Enhanced service delivery model

A second key factor believed to be fundamental in raising breastfeeding rates in the Felgate area was the enhanced midwifery capacity within the programme. The programme has sufficient midwifery resources to enable midwives to have caseloads of 70–80 women per year, as opposed to caseloads of 200, which are the average in an adjacent area. This reduced caseload has a number of important effects. First, it provides midwives with sufficient time to convey the necessary information required by the BFI to enable women to make an informed choice: 'You can sit down and really have a good talk to women about all of the different aspects. There is such a lot of information to give…it takes a lot of time'.

Second, and very importantly, Sure Start Felgate can offer intensive support to breastfeeding mothers in the critical first few weeks following birth, which is when many mothers give up. The significant difference in Sure Start Felgate is that, due to enhanced midwifery capacity, midwives can visit breastfeeding women in their homes two or three times a day to begin with; this was believed by staff to make a great difference to women who knew that they were just a phone call away. Although women could contact the local hospital, midwives stated that hospitals are generally seen as 'an alien place, a long way off'.

Mothers we spoke to confirmed that the level of support which Sure Start Felgate had offered them had been a very important factor in enabling them to start and continue breastfeeding:

> There was always someone there to talk things through – having the midwives there was very important – there was pretty much someone there every day the following week [after birth]… I feel like I've got enough support – I feel like the girls [midwives] will be there if ever I need any advice.

The fact that Sure Start Felgate midwives told women that they would offer support at any time, not only during office hours, was a key issue for some:

> I had a lot of help and support. The midwives said, "Look, we'll help you. We'll come out at all hours – in the middle of the night if we need to". And I know someone who did get a visit at night. Yeah, knowing that there's that support network gave me a lot of confidence – that's what made me give it a try.

Two women stressed the difference in terms of the level of support offered now by Sure Start Felgate, compared to that which had been available in the area previously:

> When I had [my son], there were no services or groups. I had to see a doctor for him to be weighed. I gave up breastfeeding as there was no support.

> When I was in hospital, you were pretty much left to get on with it. They would ask, "Are you breastfeeding or bottle feeding?" and, if it was the bottle,

it was, "There's a bottle, get on with it!" I was put off. There just wasn't any help.

Building relationships

Another vital benefit of having smaller caseloads was that Sure Start midwives had enough time to develop close relationships with women during their pregnancy. Women in Sure Start Felgate see the same midwife throughout their pregnancy, and see much more of her than women in non-Sure Start areas would do. Pregnant women in the area have an initial two-hour booking session at home, followed by more home visits, as well as regular clinic sessions. Another longer 90-minute session occurs at around 32 weeks. This pattern of contact is very different from that often experienced by women in mainstream services, where staff are working under pressure in busy clinics. These longer home visits enable midwives to gain more in-depth information than was possible previously. Overall, Sure Start midwives in Felgate reported that women develop trusting relationships with them which, in turn, means that they are often more willing to listen to information about breastfeeding. The centrality of the relationship between the mother and midwife in supporting breastfeeding was emphasised by several mothers we spoke to. One told us: 'I had the same midwife all the way through – it's building up that relationship, that trust, you get to know them, you can ask them questions about it [breastfeeding]', while another stated: 'It's thanks to them, my guardian angels, that I am still breastfeeding my son'.

Midwives explained that there are sometimes tensions within the close relationships they have with women, when some who go on to bottlefeed articulate the feeling that they have 'let the midwives down'. This is an uncomfortable situation for staff. For this reason, where women do decide to bottlefeed or give up breastfeeding, after having had all the Baby Friendly information, staff are careful to support women in their decision: 'We can't be in a position to know what stresses women are experiencing which might make breastfeeding too difficult a choice for them'.

Peer support

Another aspect of the programme-wide approach to promoting breastfeeding has been the establishment of the Breast Feeding Support Group and the Bump2Baby sessions for pregnant women. These are groups in which breastfeeding women can support each other, and potentially influence other mothers who have chosen bottlefeeding in the past.

Midwives reported that the programme's Bump2Baby group, in particular, has been a 'major boon'. Staff within the programme have worked hard to jettison the image of the formal parentcraft sessions by establishing this informal women-led group, with staff present 'just to keep them on the right lines'. The most influential aspect of the group, in terms of promoting breast-feeding, is having mothers who have successfully breastfed come back and talk to pregnant mothers about their experiences, the problems they have had and how they have overcome them. The aim is for mothers to see how positive the experience of breastfeeding has been for others. In addition, messages about breastfeeding are reinforced at Sure Start health clinics where videotapes about breastfeeding are always running in the background to give a 'back door' message.

Some of the mothers we spoke to had attended one or other of these groups. One mother revealed that she had only intended to breastfeed for a few days, but had gone along to the Breastfeeding Support Group and found it very helpful: 'Here I am at ten weeks still going, and it's all due to Sure Start'. Another mother talked about the variety of benefits she had gained from being able to attend the Breastfeeding Support Group over time: 'It was just nice to go. It was an ongoing thing – the group was not just about breastfeeding – you could ask about general health and there was a clinic afterwards'. One mother said simply: 'The Breastfeeding Support Group is a life saver!'

Discussion

It is clear that a programme-wide implementation of the BFI, combined with an enhanced model of service delivery and supplemented by peer support groups, was effective in significantly increasing breastfeeding rates in Sure Start Felgate, at birth and four weeks, within a relatively short period of time. The achievement is particularly impressive given the extremely low baseline figure for breastfeeding at birth in 2001, which was less than half that found amongst women of similar socioeconomic background nationally (OPCS 1995).

The effectiveness of the Baby Friendly Breastfeeding Initiative in promoting breastfeeding has been shown by two major studies which demonstrated that mothers giving birth in maternity units holding the Baby Friendly full accreditation award are significantly more likely to start breastfeeding, having taken into account individual social and demographic factors (Bartington et al. 2006, Broadfoot et al. 2005). Indeed, NICE (National Institute for Health and Clinical Excellence) (2006, p.6) has recommended that: 'All maternity care providers [whether working in hospital or in primary care] should implement an externally evaluated, structured programme that encourages breastfeeding, using the Baby Friendly Initiative (www.babyfriendly.org.uk) as a minimum standard'.

Sure Start Felgate's early success in introducing some aspects of Baby Friendly values into the community, namely a greater tolerance and willingness to provide facilities for breastfeeding locally, further supports the NESS conclusions (Latham et al. 2006) that the approach has 'started to influence services and businesses in local communities, working towards, generally, tackling the non-breastfeeding cultures' (p.41). This is an extremely important issue within a national context, where legal intervention is believed necessary to safeguard a woman's right to breastfeed in public (National Childbirth Trust 2006).

The Sure Start Felgate approach was found to increase breastfeeding rates at both birth and four weeks. This is important because, although the WHO recommends that babies are exclusively breastfed for six months, women often give up well before this, with 90 per cent of mothers who do give up saying that they had given up before they wanted to. The NESS report on breastfeeding (Latham *et al.* 2006, p.20) reported that baseline surveys in Sure Start areas showed that many mothers gave up due to:

> not being supported from birth, due to staffing issues in the hospital, or at home. Health professionals were not up to date with breastfeeding advice, they often referred to the breastfeeding counsellor. Due to busy schedules and days off, continuous support from community midwives was not available.

The enhanced midwifery service delivered by Sure Start Felgate, which allows for smaller caseloads, has been shown to provide the kind of intensive level of support for breastfeeding mothers which seems especially important in an area where there has previously been a deeply entrenched bottlefeeding culture.

The mechanisms for providing peer support adopted within the programme also appear to have played an important role for a number of women in deciding to breastfeed in the first place, and maintaining it for longer postnatally. There is significant evidence testifying to the effectiveness of peer support approaches to improving breastfeeding rates in the general population (Dennis *et al.* 2002), as well as in women from lower income backgrounds (Arlotti *et al.* 1998). In the face of cuts in funding, such an approach may be especially important for Children's Centres to pursue in terms of sustainability in the longer term.

It is clear that the achievement of significant change in breastfeeding patterns in an area where there have been deeply entrenched cultural barriers to this choice has required very high levels of both staff commitment and resourcing. The leadership of the health visitor coordinator, in introducing and driving forward the BFI, was crucial during its lengthy setting-up period. Notwithstanding the success achieved by Sure Start Felgate, especially in implementing the UNICEF BFI in a community setting, it remains unclear as to whether this success can be maintained should the levels of midwifery resource be diminished as a result of general reductions in children's centre funding. Should fewer midwives be required to manage greater caseloads in the future, the likelihood is that there will be less time to develop trusting relationships within which Baby Friendly information regarding breastfeeding can be shared and discussed. In our study, Sure Start Felgate midwives emphasised the fact that women were more likely to be influenced by the Baby Friendly information when delivered by a health professional with whom they had developed a trusting relationship. The impact of budgetary reductions on success achieved will need to be monitored closely in this key area, as well as others, to ensure that the vital gains so recently won will not be lost as local programme services are rolled out over a wider area with fewer resources.

Implications for Children's Centres

1. Improving breastfeeding rates in areas of socioeconomic disadvantage requires an intensive and integrated approach. The UNICEF BFI represents one such approach which can be successfully implemented within Children's Centres, given sufficient funding and support. Breastfeeding rates should continue to be monitored closely by Children's Centres in future years.

2. The building of trusting relationships between midwives and pregnant women seems crucial to the successful promotion of breastfeeding in areas where there are few breastfeeding role models locally. Such relationships require consistency and time to develop which, in turn, indicates the need for an enhanced midwifery provision to allow for smaller caseloads within which such relationships can be nurtured.

3. The further development of peer support mechanisms for breastfeeding women is indicated in terms of both effectiveness and sustainability.

Acknowledgements

We should like to extend our warmest thanks to those Sure Start Felgate staff who participated in this study and especially to the programme's former health visitor coordinator and current midwifery staff for their inspirational work in this area.

References

Arlotti, J.P., Cottrell, B.H., Hughes Lee, S. and Curtin, J.J. (1998) 'Breastfeeding among low-income women with and without peer support.' *Journal of Community Health Nursing 15*, 3, 163–178.

Armstrong, J.A. and Reilly, J.J. (2002) 'Breastfeeding and lowering the risk of childhood obesity.' *The Lancet 359*, 9322, 2003–2004.

Bartington, S., Griffiths, L.J., Tate, A.R. and Dezateux, C. (2006) 'Are breastfeeding rates higher among mothers delivering in Baby Friendly accredited maternity units in the UK?' *International Journal of Epidemiology 35*, 5, 1178–1186.

Bolling, K. (2006) *Infant Feeding Survey 2005: Early Results.* London: The Information Centre.

Broadfoot, M., Britten, J., Tappin, D.M. and MacKenzie, J.M. (2005) 'The Baby Friendly Hospital Initiative and breast feeding rates in Scotland.' *Archives of Disease in Childhood: Fetal and Neonatal 90*, 2, 114–116.

Dennis, C.L., Hodnett, E., Gallop, R. and Chalmers, B. (2002) 'The effect of peer support on breast-feeding duration among primiparous women: a randomized controlled trial.' *Canadian Medical Association Journal 166*, 1, 21–28.

Department for Education and Skills (2002) *A Guide for Sixth Wave Programmes.* London: DfES.

Fergusson, D.M. and Woodward, L.J. (1999) 'Breast feeding and later psychosocial adjustment.' *Paediatric and Perinatal Epidemiology 13*, 2, 144–157.

Hamlyn, B., Brooker, S., Oleinikova, K. and Wands, S. (2000) *Infant Feeding Survey.* London: DoH.

Henderson, L., Kitzinger, J. and Green, J. (2000) 'Representing infant feeding: content analysis of British media portrayals of bottle feeding and breastfeeding.' *British Medical Journal 321*, 7270, 1196–1198.

Kohner, N. (1997) *The Pregnancy Book.* London: Health Education Authority.

Latham, P., Kapoor, S., Myers, P. and Barnes, J. (2006) *Breastfeeding, Weaning and Health Eating: a Synthesis of Sure Start Local Programme Evaluation Findings.* www.ness.bbk.ac.uk/documents/synthesisReports/1241.pdf, accessed on 9 November 2006.

National Childbirth Trust (2006) *Mums Call for Breastfeeding Law.* www.nct.org.uk/media/pressrelease?prid=63, accessed on 4 December 2006.

NICE (2006) *Routine Postnatal Care of Women and their Babies.* London: DoH.

Office of Population Censuses and Surveys (1995) *Infant Feeding Survey.* London: DoH.

Robson, C. (2002) *Real World Research.* Oxford: Blackwell.

Sacker, A., Quigley, M. A. and Kelly, Y. J. (2006) 'Breastfeeding and Developmental Delay: Findings From the Millennium Cohort Study.' *Pediatrics 118*, 3, e682–689.

UNICEF Baby Friendly (2001a) 'About the Baby Friendly Initiative.' www.babyfriendly.org.uk/page.asp?page=11, accessed on 8 November 2006.

UNICEF Baby Friendly (2001b) 'Best practice in community healthcare services – the Seven Point Plan.' www.babyfriendly.org.uk/page.asp?page=71, accessed on 24 November 2006.

Villalpando, S. and Hamosh, M. (1998) 'Early and late effects of breast-feeding: does breast-feeding really matter?' *Neonatology 74*, 2, 177–191.

Yngve, A. and Sjostrom, M. (2001) 'Breastfeeding in countries of the European Union and EFTA: current and proposed recommendations, rationale, prevalence, duration and trends.' *Public Health Nutrition 4*, 2, 631–645.

Chapter 5

Evaluating the Impact of a Child Injury Prevention Project

Julie Carman, David Lamb, Ellis Friedman
and Kate Hardman

Injury in childhood is a major cause of death, ill health and disability in the UK (Department of Health 2002). Government strategy reflects concern about the death rate from accident in the general population of the United Kingdom. One of the targets set by the *Saving Lives: Our Healthier Nation* strategy (Department of Health 1999) was to: '...reduce the death rates from accidents by at least one fifth and to reduce the rate of serious injury from accidents by at least one tenth by 2010 – saving up to 12,000 lives in total'. There are, however, wide inequalities in injury mortality and morbidity experienced by different socioeconomic groups (Towner 2002), and the target was therefore aimed particularly at improving death and mortality rates amongst the worst off.

The project outlined in this chapter was intended specifically to address prevention of injury to children from lower socioeconomic groups and embraced the cross-government ambitions of the *Delivering Choosing Health* agenda (Department of Health 2005) in helping children and young people lead healthier lives by applying the key principles of informed choice for all, personalised support to make healthier choices and working in partnership to make health everyone's business. By providing information and advice across a locality, and targeted intervention via the Home Safety Equipment Scheme (HSES) to parents requiring additional support, it also supported the key outcomes of *Every Child Matters* (Department for Education and Skills 2003), particularly 'staying safe', by helping parents and carers to ensure early intervention and effective protection from unintentional injury.

Numerous researchers have shown that unintentional childhood injuries are strongly associated with poverty (Towner *et al.* 2005). The social class gradient for deaths due to injuries is steeper than for any other cause of childhood death (Dowswell and Towner 2002; Laing and Logan 1999; Roberts and Power 1996). A study of the period 1989–1992 (the most recent located) found that a child born into a social class 5 family was five times more likely to have an unintentional injury, and 16 times more likely to suffer a home fire accident, than a child born into a social class 1 family (Towner *et al.* 2005). It is estimated that more that half the deaths among children aged under five occur in the home (Towner and Dowswell 2001). A recent report published jointly by the Audit Commission and Healthcare Commission (2007) reiterated the significant burden placed by unintentional injury to children on the NHS, local government, and the families and individuals affected. Although the overall number of deaths has fallen, the report shows that there are persistent and widening differences between socioeconomic groups. Access to clear information about the availability of safety equipment, its cost and the process of installing it may be barriers to implementing home safety practices, particularly among low income and non-white ethnic minority families (DiGuieseppi and Roberts 2000; Mulvaney and Kendrick 2004).

Currently there is reasonable evidence that the provision of low-cost safety equipment, in conjunction with safety counselling, can result in increases in safety practices and the reduction of hazards in the home (Nilson 2004). However, the effect on actual injury rates is less clear. One recently published study based in deprived areas of Nottingham (Watson *et al.* 2005) has examined the provision and fitting of safety equipment, free of charge, in conjunction with safety advice and information. This randomised controlled study found medically attended injuries to be significantly higher in the intervention group. A possible explanation for this was poor penetration of the intervention: only 35 per cent of the eligible families invited to participate in the trial did so. Families with higher levels of disadvantage may have been less likely to participate. Furthermore, only 38 per cent of the intervention arm actually received the safety equipment which would limit the potential for the intervention to show an effect. The findings of the Action on Children's Accidents Project (ACAP) intervention described in this chapter were, however, contrary to Watson's study because, although the absolute injury rates were higher in the intervention group, the decrease in injury rates was greater in the intervention group than in the comparison group.

Nilson's systematic review of community injury prevention work (Nilson 2004) suggests that hundreds of community-based injury prevention programmes have been implemented since the mid 1970s, but few have been evaluated rigorously. This has led to a lack of consensus as to whether it is an effective strategy for reducing injuries. Towner and Dowswell (2001) also recommend that community-based injury prevention should be evaluated and the benefits of different approaches be debated. This chapter contributes to this debate by describing an evaluation of a child injury prevention project in deprived localities. It aims to add to the existing knowledge base about child injury prevention by describing how the project was set up, the results of the quantitative evaluation to date, and by estimating the cost-effectiveness of the project.

Background

Burnley, Pendle and Rossendale Primary Care Trust (PCT) serves a population of approximately 250,000, of whom around 15,000 (6%) are aged under five. Based on the *Index of Multiple Deprivation* scores (Office of the Deputy Prime Minister 2004), Burnley borough is ranked 37th most deprived of the 354 local authorities in England, and Pendle and Rossendale are ranked 71st and 92nd respectively. The PCT population includes a relatively large Pakistani community, with 11.5 per cent of the Pendle and 4.3 per cent of the Burnley population being Pakistani (Office for National Statistics 2001). Local Accident and Emergency (A&E) data indicate that, every year, one in three children under five years of age living in more disadvantaged wards is attending A&E with an injury. This is higher than the national average of around one in five children attending A&E.

The project

The overall aim of the project was to reduce the number of children under five years of age attending A&E with an unintentional injury. There were three specific aspects:

1. A targeted HSES operating in Sure Start wards. The funding for this aspect of the project came from Sure Start programmes and neighbourhood renewal funding monies and could therefore only be delivered in the most disadvantaged wards. A service level agreement is in place to deliver the HSES to 200 family homes in each Sure Start programme area per year.

2. A population-wide outreach and education approach to child injury prevention delivered by the ACAP team via a multi-agency network across the PCT locality.

3. Follow-up of families after an unintentional home injury to prevent further injuries. An A&E slip was returned to the local health visitor who offered the families safety advice and the opportunity to be referred to the ACAP Home Safety Equipment Scheme if they were in the eligible areas.

The ACAP team

The Action on Children's Accidents Project was managed as part of the public health directorate of Burnley, Pendle and Rossendale PCT. In 2001, the ACAP coordinator developed and began delivering the project in the first Sure Start programme area. As further local Sure Start programmes were established, additional team members were recruited. The team increased to include the coordinator, three project workers and an administration officer. The team has a mix of skills including: health promotion, business, media and communications, and nursing. In addition, team members have undertaken specific home safety training offered by the Royal Society for the Prevention of Accidents (RoSPA) and the Child Accident Prevention Trust (CAPT).

The Home Safety Equipment Scheme

The HSES was introduced in phases over the period 2001 to 2003 to Sure Start areas across Burnley and Pendle. The remaining more affluent wards form a non-intervention comparison group. Figure 5.1 describes the phased introduction of the scheme.

Parents of children aged under five years who were registered with the designated Sure Start areas were offered a home safety visit by a project worker from the ACAP team. A simple referral form carried by health visitors, midwives, Sure Start outreach workers and social workers was completed and returned to the ACAP office. The team then contacted the family to arrange a mutually convenient time to carry out a home visit. Health visitors notified of a child's accident by the health visitor liaison team at the local hospital can ensure families living in Sure Start areas are offered the HSES.

At the visit, home safety was discussed and a pack of leaflets, information and small items of equipment were left with the family (Figure 5.2).

Using a checklist, parents were given advice on how to prevent falls, burns and scalds, poisoning and other home injuries. Arrangements were then made for larger items of equipment (Figure 5.3) to be fitted by trained technicians from a local care and repair agency.

The average total cost of the package provided is £165 (including time and travel expenses for the ACAP project worker and the fitters, and cost of equipment and fitting). Families were asked to contribute £5 towards this cost.

October 2001	PENDLE Sure Start (Bradley and Whitefield Wards)
August 2002	WATERBRIDGE Sure Start (Waterside, Vivary Bridge, Horsfield Wards)
January 2003	SOUTH WEST BURNLEY Sure Start (Barclay, Bank Hall, Coal Clough, Trinity, Gawthorpe and Fulledge Wards)
February 2003	BRIERFIELD AND WALVERDEN Sure Start (Brierfield and Walverden Wards)
October 2003	DUKE BAR AND BURNLEY WOOD Sure Start (wards in the Duke Bar and Burnley Wood area)
March 2004	Evaluation

Figure 5.1 Phased introduction of the HSES to Sure Start programme areas in Burnley and Pendle

1. Bath mat
2. Harness and reins
3. Cupboard locks
4. Corner cushions
5. Adhesive multipurpose lock
6. Plug socket covers

Figure 5.2 Items left with families at ACAP project worker's visit

1. Safety gates
2. Fireguards
3. Ten-year smoke alarm
4. Kitchen cupboard locks
5. Safety film for glass door panels

Figure 5.3 Range of items fitted by home care and repair technicians (depending on layout of home and age of children)

Population-wide outreach and education

The ACAP team delivered home safety talks across the PCT locality in a number of settings, including Sure Start groups, nurseries, play groups, teen-parent and community groups, to raise awareness of how easily home injuries can occur and how they can be prevented. In addition to information leaflets, the team provided tea-towels printed with safety messages, videos, CDs, games and activity sheets. Resources were obtained and developed by the team to enable messages to be shared in a number of ways with families who may not have English as a first language or who have low levels of literacy. The team provided training days on accident prevention for PCT staff and early years workers.

A SAFE network (Safety Awareness for Everyone) was set up by the ACAP project coordinator which provided population-wide safety events in local shopping centres across the PCT locality. SAFE events were themed around child safety week, firework safety, seasonal safety, cycle safety, road safety and supporting school and community events. The network is made up of stakeholder agencies including representation from:

- Fire and Rescue Service
- Road Policing Unit

- health visitor liaison (from the acute trust)
- Network Rail
- health visitors
- school nurses
- local Sure Start programmes
- Lancashire Partnership for Road Safety
- Safer Travel Unit
- Leisure Trust
- East Lancashire Business Partnership
- Ambulance Trust
- voluntary and community groups.

Evaluation

Method

Data on attendances at A&E by children under the age of five following an injury were extracted for intervention and comparison wards for the four-year period 1999–2000 to 2003–2004 (i.e. two years prior to the first wave intervention to six months after the last wave). The data analysed were from the A&E database at the East Lancashire Hospitals Trust and included postcode of residence and type of incident. Incidents defined as 'minor ailments' were excluded from the analysis. The Office for National Statistics publishes data matching postcodes to electoral wards. Using this information, the postcodes of the children attending A&E were allocated to their electoral ward of residence. For each ward in Burnley and Pendle, the number of children attending A&E was divided by the population of children aged under five to calculate the percentage of children attending A&E. In addition, to make some assessment of the potential cost benefits of the programme, information on injury reduction following the implementation of the project was used in conjunction with national estimates of the cost of treating an injury in hospital to calculate the costs associated with delivery of the programme.

Results

ATTENDANCE FIGURES AT A&E

Tables 5.1 and 5.2 show the proportion of children attending Burnley General Hospital A&E Department. The population of children aged under five was estimated for each year of the analysis. A&E attendance figures show a greater decrease in the number of children under five from the intervention wards attending A&E due to an injury than from the comparison wards.

Table 5.1 Number of Burnley and Pendle children aged under five attending A&E at Burnley General Hospital (excluding minor ailments)

Year	Sure Start area	Other areas	Total
2000–2001	2012	1099	3111
2001–2002	1982	1175	3157
2002–2003	1732	1057	2789
2003–2004	1551	900	2451
Percentage reduction	22.9%	18.1%	21.2%

Table 5.1 shows that between 2000 and 2004 there was a reduction in A&E attendance by Burnley and Pendle children aged under five. The rate of reduction was greater in wards where there had been a Sure Start intervention than in other areas of Burnley and Pendle. There was a reduction of 21 per cent in the total number of under fives attending A&E in 2003–2004 compared to 2000–2001, before the project began, and a faster rate of decline in A&E attendances by children in the Sure Start areas compared to the other wards. In 2000–2001 the relative risk of a child in a Sure Start area attending A&E compared to the non-intervention areas was 1.3 (95% confidence interval (CI) 1.2–1.4) whereas in 2003–2004, the relative risk had decreased to 1.2 (95% CI 1.1–1.3). Although children in a Sure Start area still showed a higher probability of attending A&E than children elsewhere in the two boroughs, the gap had narrowed.

In 2000–2001, children from the two areas in the study accounted for 3111 A&E attendances. By 2003–2004 this had decreased to 2451, a difference of 660 (21%). In the absence of any other obvious factors, it is reasonable to attribute most of the reduction to ACAP. ACAP has had a direct influence in the Sure Start areas through the provision of household equipment and adaptations. The project also, by means of safety events and publicity campaigns, has raised awareness of safety issues. Some of the reduction in A&E attendances by children outside the Sure Start area may also be attributed to ACAP. Table 5.2 shows that the reduction in the proportion of children attending A&E was greater among those resident in the Sure Start areas (7.4%) than elsewhere in Burnley and Pendle (4.0%). The gap between the two areas has narrowed.

Table 5.2 Proportion of Burnley and Pendle children aged under five attending
A&E at Burnley General Hospital (excluding minor ailments)

Year	Sure Start area	Other areas
2000–2001	36.0%	28.2%
2001–2002	35.6%	31.4%
2002–2003	35.0%	31.9%
2003–2004	28.6%	24.2%

COST-EFFECTIVENESS

The Transport Research Laboratory estimates the average cost of hospital treatment following an event in the home which results in an unintentional injury of slight severity to be £3920 (based on 1994 prices) (Transport Research Laboratory 1996). RoSPA estimates this to represent just over £5000 at 2001 prices (RoSPA 2003). In the intervention wards, there were 660 fewer A&E attendances in 2003–2004 by children aged under five compared with 2000–2001. Assuming the average cost of each attendance to have been £5000, a reduction of this magnitude saved the local health economy £3,300,000. It is not feasible, however, to attribute the entire reduction to ACAP. It is more reasonable to hypothesise that the introduction of ACAP led to between 30 and 80 per cent of the reduction in A&E attendances in the Sure Start area. Knowledge of ACAP extended beyond the Sure Start area and there is some evidence that the project raised awareness of the importance of safety in the home in other areas of Burnley and Pendle. It can be assumed that ACAP may, therefore, have been directly responsible for up to 30 per cent of the reduction in A&E attendances in those areas. Using these figures it is possible to suggest a range of realistic estimates of the financial savings resulting from ACAP.

Calculation 1

The 'high influence' hypothesis suggests that ACAP was responsible for 80 per cent of the reduction in attendances in Sure Start areas (where HSES was provided) and 30 per cent in those areas which did not receive the intervention but were exposed to population-wide events. On this basis, the savings amounted to £2,256,000. To date, the project has cost £359,000 to deliver. The total saving is therefore £1,900,000.

Calculation 2

The 'low influence' hypothesis suggests that ACAP influenced only 30 per cent of the reduction in A&E attendances in the Sure Start area and none in the other areas. This suggests a saving of £690,000 dropping to £331,000 when the costs of delivering the project are subtracted.

Comparing the effect with an area receiving no intervention

A preliminary examination of A&E attendance by children aged under five in the neighbouring Borough of Rossendale, where no intervention had taken place, suggests a continuing rise in attendance.

Views of service users

A users' satisfaction survey was carried out with families who had accessed the HSES. Comments were extremely positive, and any suggestions for improvement were considered and implemented, if it was possible to do so. Of 100 service users recently approached as part of the evaluation across the five areas, 95 per cent said they felt their children were a lot safer since they had received advice and had the safety equipment fitted, while the remainder felt their children were a little safer. Typical comments were:

> It's good to be spoken to on a level and not looked down on. Thank you.

> Great value for money.

> Very happy. Excellent service.

> Fantastic – I'm a first time mum and I didn't know anything about safety.

> I tell everyone that comes to the house – it's brilliant.

> The fitter was really helpful.

Discussion

Injuries are one of the major causes of death and serious morbidity in young children. The incidence is higher in disadvantaged areas. This ACAP project, which has provided outreach and education across the locality in addition to a targeted home safety equipment scheme accessed by 1234 families, has had a measurable impact on reducing attendance due to injury at the local A&E department. The relatively low proportion of eligible families who received the intervention in Watson *et al.*'s (2005) study may have limited the potential for the impact to show effect. In our project, the proportion of eligible families who accessed the HSES was relatively high: 1234 families, which we estimate to represent over 50 per cent of eligible families.

It is important to recognise that this project was not established as a randomised controlled trial. However, since several wards in Burnley and Pendle were not eligible to receive the ACAP service, these wards served as a comparison group. The intervention wards generally experienced higher levels of socioeconomic disadvantage than the comparison area. This is because funding for the HSES project came from Sure Start and neighbourhood renewal monies which could be delivered only in the most disadvantaged wards. However, assuming that the intervention wards contain a higher proportion of 'harder to reach' groups, we would expect a reduction in accident rates to be more difficult to achieve than in the comparison wards. This adds weight to argument that the greater decline in attendance rates observed in the intervention wards was due to the project.

In carrying out the evaluation, it was also important to recognise that families in the comparison group of wards, who were not eligible for the HSES, may have received home safety advice and education via the national and local media, word of mouth and the local safety events. The Sure Start families may also have received other interventions and support in addition to ACAP that the non-intervention families will not have received. Both these factors may have influenced the findings.

The quality of the data from A&E and the current availability of information around the costing of an injury are not entirely robust, but are the best that could be obtained at the time. Indeed, a further objective of the project has been work to improve and refine data collection relating to children's injuries at the local A&E department.

Over the period 1999–2000 to 2003–2004, evaluation of the ACAP project has shown a decrease in A&E attendance, in particular from children living in the intervention areas. Costing the potential benefits to the local health economy has shown the project's cost-effectiveness, as well as contributing to the evidence available on what works in reducing childhood injuries. In addition, we have found evidence of a narrowing of the gap between the Sure Start and non-intervention areas.

Conclusion

Our approach to reducing childhood injuries, which is transferable to other settings, demonstrated a local beneficial effect. It is likely that similar positive outcomes could be achieved nationally and internationally.

By providing a coordinated approach combining advice, education and environmental modification, and working with parents to help them make their homes safer, tangible benefits have been achieved. This is providing real health gains for the local population, reducing the health gap and health inequalities, and ensuring children can reach their full potential at home and at school.

Authors' note

This chapter was originally published in *Community Practitioner*, volume 79, pp.188–192 with the same title and is reprinted with minor amendments and with the permission of the publishers.

Acknowledgements

The authors wish to acknowledge Mima Cattan, Mike Hayes, Bob Harbin and Tim Mansfield for their helpful comments on the manuscript.

References

Audit Commission and Healthcare Commission (2007) *Better Safe than Sorry: Preventing Unintentional Injury to Children.* London: Audit Commission.

Department for Education and Skills (2003) *Every Child Matters.* London: HMSO.

Department of Health (1999) *Saving Lives: Our Healthier Nation.* London: HMSO.

Department of Health (2002) *Preventing Accidental Injury – Priorities for Action.* (Report for the Accidental Injury Task Force to the Chief Medical Officer.) London: DoH.

Department of Health (2005) *Delivering Choosing Health: Making Healthier Choices Easier.* London: DoH.

DiGuieseppi, C. and Roberts, I.G. (2000) 'Individual-level injury prevention strategies in the clinical setting.' *Future Child 10,* 1, 53–82.

Dowswell, T. and Towner, E. (2002) 'Social deprivation and the prevention of unintentional injury in childhood: a systematic review.' *Health Education Research 17,* 2, 221–237.

Laing, G. and Logan, S. (1999) 'Patterns of unintentional injury in childhood and their relation to socio-economic factors.' *Public Health 113,* 6, 291–294.

Mulvaney, C. and Kendrick, D. (2004) 'Engagement in safety practices to prevent home injuries in preschool children among white and non-white ethnic minority families.' *Injury Prevention 10,* 6, 375–378.

Nilson, P. (2004) 'What makes community based injury prevention work? In search of evidence of effectiveness.' *Injury Prevention 10,* 5, 268–274.

Office for National Statistics (2001) *Census of Population.* London: ONS.

Office of the Deputy Prime Minister (2004) *The English Indices of Deprivation.* London: ODPM.

Roberts, I. and Power, C. (1996) 'Does the decline in child injury mortality vary by social class? A comparison of class specific mortality in 1981 and 1991.' *British Medical Journal 313,* 784–786.

Royal Society for the Prevention of Accidents (RoSPA) (2003) 'Costs and causes of accidents.' *City and Guilds Introducing Home Safety,* Issue 3.

Towner, E. (2002) *The Prevention of Childhood Injury: Background Paper Prepared for the Accidental Injury Task Force.* Newcastle: Department of Child Health.

Towner, E. and Dowswell, T. (2001) *What Works to Prevent Unintentional Injury Amongst Children?* (Report prepared for the Health Development Agency, London.) Newcastle: Department of Child Health, University of Newcastle.

Towner, E., Dowswell, T., Errington, G., Burkes, M. and Towner, J. (2005) *Injuries in Children Aged 0–14 and Inequalities.* (Report prepared for the Health Development Agency, London.) Newcastle: Department of Child Health, University of Newcastle.

Transport Research Laboratory (1996) *Valuation of Home Accidents: A Comparative Review of Home and Road Accidents.* TRL Report 225.

Watson, M., Kendrick, D., Coupland, C., Woods, A., Futers, D. and Robinson, J. (2005) 'Providing child safety equipment to prevent injuries: randomised controlled trial.' *British Medical Journal 330,* 178–181.

Chapter 6

Training for Language-enriched Pre-school Settings

Carol Potter and Sharon Hodgson

The overall goal for Sure Start Local Programmes was:

> to work with parents-to-be, parents and children to promote the physical, intellectual and social development of babies and young children – particularly those who are disadvantaged – so that they can flourish at home and when they get to school, and hereby break the cycle of disadvantage for the current generation of young children. (Department for Education and Skills 2002, p.3)

An important approach to securing such an outcome was the provision of 'good quality play, learning and childcare experiences for children' (Department for Education and Skills 2002, p.4). Assessing the quality of such environments has therefore been an important aspect of local evaluations. Sure Start Hinton (pseudonym) asked Durham University to undertake an evaluation of the quality of their play settings provided in 2002 and again in 2003, using the Early Childhood Environmental Rating Scale – Revised (ECERS–R, Harms, Clifford and Cryer 1998) which assesses quality in seven areas, namely: space and furnishings, personal and care routines, language-reasoning, activities, interaction, programme structure, and parents and staff.

The results showed that there was an improvement in the quality of play in 2003, with sessions observed rated 'good' in nearly all areas measured by the ECERS–R. However, scores in the area of language and reasoning were relatively low, as has been the pattern in a number of other studies, both within the UK and abroad (Bryant, Peisner-Feinberg and Clifford 1993; Potter 2005). There appear to be a number of possible explanations for the difficulty in providing high quality communication environments in pre-school settings, relating to unfavourable staffing ratios and the necessity for staff to engage in a range of tasks, many of which are not directly child-related (Kontos 1999).

As a result of these findings, Sure Start Hinton undertook a review of the possible ways in which it could improve the quality of its language and communication environments across the programme in close collaboration with its speech and language therapist. It was decided to pilot an intensive, practice-based training course for key staff, focusing on language enhancement within pre-school settings.

The programme's speech and language therapist designed an innovative 12-week Adult–Child Interaction (ACI) training course for five trained nursery nurse staff, four of whom were working in an Early Years Group, which admits children aged two to four years, and one of whom was based in the programme's day care provision, which caters for children three years and under.

The ACI training course consisted of the following components:

- six two-hour introductory sessions: these were included to ensure that the background knowledge of all staff was similar on beginning the following six training sessions

- six two-hour training sessions (see Table 6.1), to take place every other week, during which video clips of staff's own practice would be viewed

- six follow-up work-based support visits to each setting by the speech and language therapy trainer to take place on alternate weeks to the training sessions.

Table 6.1 ACI training schedule

Session	Content
Session 1	Expectations and communication
Session 2	Adjusting the way you talk
Session 3	Play
Session 4	Attention and listening
Session 5	Turn-taking and group facilitation
Session 6	Praise and encouragement

Methodology

Since Durham University had carried out the original quality of play evaluation which led to the development of the ACI training, Sure Start Hinton also asked the University to evaluate this second stage of its work. Research questions for the evaluation of the ACI course were as follows:

- Can the ACI course change how adults talk with children? (The nature of the verbal prompts which adults use with children can enhance or inhibit their speech and language development.)

- Following training, do staff provide more frequent, high quality communication opportunities in everyday sessions?

- Do interactions between adults and children become more child-led following training?

- What are the staff perceptions of the training? What was most/least helpful? Why? What do the staff think could be done differently?

To answer these questions, we used the following research methods:

- video clips of staff interacting with children before and after the training

- observations at staff training sessions

- pre- and post-training interviews with speech and language therapist

- pre-training focus group with nursery nurse staff

- post-training interviews with nursery nurse staff.

Videotape analysis

Five minutes of videotape of nursery nurses interacting with one child and with a group of children were taken before and after the training. The young age of the children in the day care unit made it inappropriate for group activities to take place in that setting. Videotape was analysed using a system developed by Law, Barnett and Kot (1999), which allows for a detailed analysis of adult and child interactions. It looks specifically at the following:

- *Discourse structure* (adult and child). Who begins interactions and how is the interaction maintained?

- *Communicative function* (adult only). What communication is being used for – to ask questions, to direct, to continue a topic?

- *Linguistic behaviour* (adult only). How do adults help children to consolidate and develop their use of language, by providing word mapping opportunities, for example?

Videotapes were transcribed and coded using this framework and then analysed using the Statistical Package for Social Sciences (SPSS).

Findings

Focus groups and staff interviews

Before the ACI course, staff training in language and communication was limited. Sure Start Hinton nursery nurses had attended different initial training courses and so the content of their training varied to some extent. However, it was clear that none of the courses attended had provided staff with any in-depth training in the area of language and communication and how to promote it. One nursery nurse said:

> You don't get a lot of that in your training so I didn't have a great big knowledge of communication and language and development – what stages they were at and when – so I didn't have a very good knowledge of that.

Staff felt that this lack of training in the crucial area of communication development caused them significant difficulties in their everyday practice. This was especially the case in their catchment area where a large number of children required significant support with language development.

After the ACI course, it was clear that it had brought about important changes, both to staff understanding of language and communication development and, critically, to their practice in this area. All staff believed that their understanding of the development of language and communication in the early years had increased following the course. Some of the comments from staff were as follows:

> [I didn't know] what stages children were at and when – so I didn't have a very good knowledge of that – so the course was helpful.

> I think I've got a better understanding of speech development.

After the course, staff talked about their new-found understanding of what they could do to promote children's communication better. They gave examples of how they needed to change how they spoke to children to encourage better communication from them. More significantly perhaps, it was also clear from videotaped material that staff had begun to change their practice in important ways.

Reducing the use of questions

An important goal of the ACI course was to help staff reflect on the strategies they regularly used to promote interaction with children. The use of questions was one area for discussion since it is known that the over-use of questions with young children can serve to inhibit language development (Wells 1985). After the ACI course had finished, we found that one of the most frequently mentioned areas of learning highlighted by staff was the need to reduce the number of questions they asked children:

> Not asking questions of children – not putting pressure on children.
>
> Not questioning as much.

Staff not only understood the importance of particular approaches but they also felt that they were now using them in their everyday practice. For example, one member of staff said:

> I do question but not as much and I try not to make it such a dead end question.

Having said this, the experience of implementing new strategies clearly takes time as well as effort and reflection. We asked staff to tell us about their experience of trying to put the new approaches into practice.

> I think you do have to think about it – obviously because you're used to asking questions and sometimes you do do it and you think "Aahh", now that you know that and you do get the dead end response from the child and you do think "Oh – I shouldn't have asked that question" so I'm still learning from any little mistakes…but I know now whereas before I would not have realised you know…

Using pauses

Another strategy introduced during the course was the use of pausing more during interactions with children. Once again videotaped material was introduced to enable staff to reflect on this area of their practice during the training. Staff talked about the impact of this learning on their approach after the course was finished:

> Definitely, learning to pause, giving the child the chance to speak – not feeling that just because there's a silence I've got to fill it.
>
> Maybe pausing a lot more – not thinking "Oh no there's a silence – I've got to fill it with something – do something".

Staff mentioned that they had already used these approaches in their daily interactions with children.

> At first – I was very conscious of it – thinking "I must pause here" or "I mustn't ask a question" – where now – it's just everyday life – I just do it now.

Simplifying language

Another course strategy taught on the ACI course, which staff said had a particular impact on their thinking, was the need to simplify the language used with some children.

> Cutting down the amount of language – going down to a two-word sentence rather than a three…not to say things like – "Would you like to hang your coat up?" – although that sounds more polite – you know "coat on peg" – it gets the message over.

Staff gave examples of how they had begun to use these new strategies in their everyday practice, noting the positive response on children's language:

> We're getting a lot of response because we've started to shorten what we say to them – two or three words put together.

Staff commented on the positive impact which changes in their practice seemed to have had on children in the areas of concentration, understanding and use of language:

> It's been really positive – we're getting a lot of response.

> I think it's made a big change for the children – allowing the children to take the lead – we've empowered them really.

> I've had language from some children who I would not have thought were capable of describing their pictures.

These are very positive findings since they indicate that children were beginning to benefit from the changes in adult language behaviour in terms of understanding and expression.

Videotape analysis

For analysis of videotaped data, we transcribed and coded five consecutive minutes of ACI (that is five pairs) taken at random from a longer interaction, before and after the ACI training course. The same process was undertaken when coding videotape of four of the same staff working with a small group of children before and after training. We then counted the number of verbal initiations, verbal responses, questions and language word-mapping opportunities (that is occasions when adults built on what children had said by providing additional concepts). In total 1984 adult and child utterances were coded. Coding was undertaken by two raters with an independent agreement of 84 per cent.

Verbal initiations

Research has shown that in order for children to become effective communicators, it is vital that they have extensive experience of leading interactions with adults (Ward 1999). In order for them to do this, adults must be prepared and able to allow children to initiate more often. If children only have experience of responding to what adults say in their early years, this can result in poorer language development. A key question for the research therefore was: did adults begin fewer interactions after the ACI training than before?

On average, adults did begin *significantly fewer* interactions with individual children after the training than before. This difference was statistically significant (p=0.04), meaning that the difference in staff behaviour in this area after the training was unlikely to be due to chance. In effect, this means that one-to-one interactions were more child-led after the training than before. This change in language behaviour is likely to be strongly linked with staff's increased use of pausing, discussed above, since this would provide additional time for children to begin a verbal interaction.

Figures 6.1 and 6.2 show the average proportion of interactions started by adults and children before and after training. Figure 6.3 shows the number of verbal initiations in one-to-one interactions used by each member of staff before and after training.

The average number of initiations was 30 at Time 1 with a standard deviation (SD) of 10.9. At Time 2, the average was 15 with an SD of 6.5. After training, not only was the frequency of staff-initiated talk halved, but there was also less difference between members of staff in terms of their number of

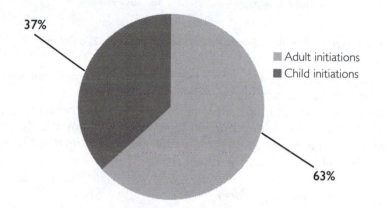

Figure 6.1 Proportion of adult and child initiations in one-to-one interactions before training

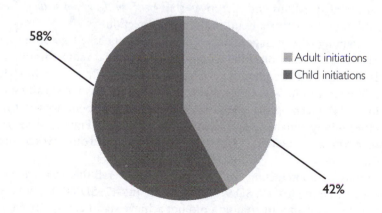

Figure 6.2 Proportion of adult and child initiations in one-to-one interactions after training

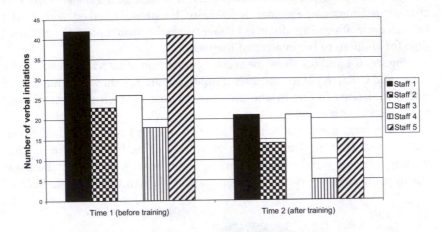

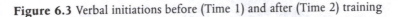

Figure 6.3 Verbal initiations before (Time 1) and after (Time 2) training

initiations. This is important because it means that there was more consistency across the staff team in how staff were interacting with children.

There were fewer adult initiations in the group setting after training but this difference did not achieve statistical significance (p=0.06). Clearly, there had been change in the same direction, a reduction in adult initiated speech, even though not a statistically significant change.

Asking questions/directing children

We explored whether staff asked fewer questions after ACI training and found that overall adults used significantly fewer questions/directives in one-to-one interactions after the training than before. There was no significant difference in the number of questions and directives staff used *in the group setting* after training, although there was a trend in the right direction.

Before training, the average number of times adults asked questions or directed children in one-to-one interactions (asked them to do something) was 34 (SD 16.4). After the training, the average across the five members of staff had gone down to 13 (SD 7.3). Once again, this difference was statistically significant (p=0.04), meaning that there was a change in staff behaviour in this area after the training which was unlikely to be due to chance. Figure 6.4 shows the differences in the same staff members' use of questions and directives before and after training.

When staff were interacting with a small group, overall there were fewer questions after training (n=19; SD 9.9) than before (n=47; SD 20.04) but the difference before and after the training did not achieve statistical significance. However, again, it is important to note that results showed a tendency towards improvement.

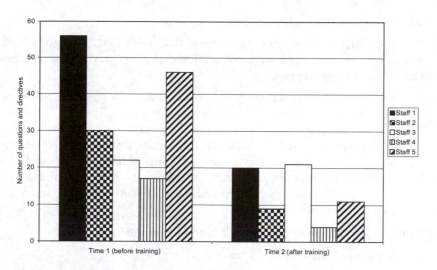

Figure 6.4 Use of questions and directives with individual children before (Time 1) and after (Time 2) training

Language learning opportunities

Providing extensive 'word mapping' opportunities is an extremely important aspect of language enhancement. A word learning or mapping opportunity occurs when adults add or scaffold new words on to what children have said. The following is an example of a word mapping opportunity:

> Child: Boat!
>
> Adult: Yes, it's a big red boat.

Snow and Paez (2004) stated that 'Vocabulary and word knowledge are crucial to literacy achievement. In fact the best single predictor of reading success is vocabulary size' (p.115). Studies have shown that children from less advantaged areas have much smaller vocabularies than children from more affluent areas (Hart and Risley 1995) and this difference predicts poorer academic achievement. It is by extending what children say, through adding new concepts and ideas, that staff have the opportunity to increase the size of children's vocabulary, which in turn can improve later success with reading. A key question for this study was therefore: did adults offer more word learning opportunities after their training than before?

Over the whole staff group, adults did not offer more word mapping opportunities after training in individual interactions with children nor in the group situation. Some staff did offer more word learning opportunities after training whilst others offered fewer. The ACI course did address the issue of scaffolding additional language on to children's own words but clearly this is a complex area and may well require additional teaching and reflection to enable staff to take on board more fully the key aspects of the approach.

Training approaches: what worked

It was clear that the viewing of video clips of staff's own practice, together with work-based support visits, were powerful and effective teaching approaches. One nursery nurse commented:

> You go on a training course – you pick the leaflets up – you listen to the presentations – they're usually done over a half day, a one day and filed away – here you had ongoing training – you had a period of time – you had key aims and it was work-based – it was practical – it made sense – to deliver it in this way with the follow-up every week – personally relating it to children – watching the videos that you understood because it was your performance – it was the child's interaction – it was real…it made sense to do it the way we've done it.

Examples of staff comments relating to the use of video clips were:

> It was good…it worked – it really did.

> Watching the videos that you…it was real – it just made sense.

The use of a work-based approach within the ACI course was a particularly innovative aspect in a course of this nature and believed by the staff concerned to be a critical one:

> The course wouldn't work without it.

> I don't think the theory side would have made enough sense without the practical input.

During support sessions, when the speech and language therapist visited settings, staff valued the opportunity to ask for her comments on their attempts to translate theory into practice, as well as to ask questions about the implementation of approaches as they arose in the practice context.

Discussion

The ACI training programme has been shown to be effective in a number of important ways. Staff demonstrated an increased understanding of language and communication development as well as better ways of facilitating ACI. This greater understanding led to some significant changes in their own practice, leading to improvements in the language and communication environment being offered to children. During and after training, staff were better able to reflect critically on their own language behaviour and adapt it in their everyday practice setting. The fact that, overall, adults were leading interactions less after training than before is a very positive finding. It suggests that the training had been successful in enabling staff to change a very important aspect of their language behaviour at the level of one-to-one interaction. Less dramatic results for the group setting may well indicate the increased difficulty of changing language behaviour when working with more than one child, although it is clear that adults were beginning to do so.

Findings from this study seem especially important in the light of current knowledge about the importance of language and communication development in the early years. It is now well accepted that both the number and quality of young children's linguistic interactions are clearly linked to outcomes later on (Hart and Risley 1995; Siraj-Blatchford *et al.* 2002). This is largely due to the close links that are widely believed to exist between spoken language and literacy skills (Catts and Kamhi 1986; Hatcher and Hulme 1999; Snow 1991). The finding that children living in areas of socioeconomic disadvantage are much more likely to experience language delay than other children (Locke, Ginsborg and Peers 2002) is therefore especially concerning since it means that these children are much more likely to achieve less at school because their literacy skills are also likely to be delayed. It is therefore especially important that children living in areas of disadvantage experience language-enriched pre-school environments. Locke *et al.*'s (2002) assertion that little is being done to increase nursery staff's knowledge of the development of spoken language is therefore of particular concern.

This study has demonstrated that a practice-based approach to staff development has significant potential for improving the ability of nursery nurses to enhance the language and communication environment of children in early years settings. It is hoped that the government's current emphasis on improving quality in the early years will recognise the importance of modifying the curriculum for initial nursery nurse training to include vital additional material on language development and approaches to language enhancement in pre-school settings. With regard to post-training staff development, it is important that attention is paid not only to what is taught but also to how it is taught. In this study, the use of video clips and work-based support sessions was viewed by staff as being crucial to achieving some impressive levels of practice change.

Implications for Children's Centres

A long-term investment in the skills and knowledge of *all* Early Years staff and professionals with regard to language development and enhancement should be considered. Specifically this means the following:

1. Language outcomes at the end of the pre-school period should remain a target within the Children's Centre agenda, since language skills are demonstrably an important predictor of academic achievement.

2. Much greater emphasis should be placed on how to promote effective ACI in both initial Early Years training courses and later professional development. The use of video and work-based learning

appear to be promising approaches to the delivery of teaching and learning in this key area.

3. Speech and language therapy advice and services remain integral to the achievement of the above goals and steps should be taken to strengthen and build upon existing partnerships between Children's Centres and the local PCTs.

References

Bryant, D.M., Peisner-Feinberg, E. and Clifford, R. (1993) *Evaluation of Public Preschool Programs in North Carolina.* Chapel Hill, NC: Frank Porter Graham Center, University of North Carolina, ED 373 882.

Catts, H.W. and Kamhi, A.G. (1986) 'The linguistic basis of reading disorders: implications for the speech-language pathologist.' *Language, Speech and Hearing Services in Schools 17,* 329–341.

Department for Education and Skills (2002) *A Guide For Sixth Wave Programmes.* London: DfES (Sure Start Unit).

Harms, T., Clifford, R.M. and Cryer, D. (1998) *Early Childhood Environment Rating Scale – Revised Edition.* London and New York, NY: Teachers College Press.

Hart, B. and Risley, T.R. (1995) *Meaningful Differences in the Everyday Experience of Young American Children.* Baltimore, MD: Paul Brookes.

Hatcher, P.J. and Hulme, C. (1999) 'Phonemes, rhymes and intelligence as predictors of children's responsiveness to remedial reading instruction: evidence from a longitudinal study.' *Journal of Experimental Child Psychology 72,* 130–153.

Kontos, S. (1999) 'Preschool teachers' talk, roles and activity settings during free play.' *Early Childhood Research Quarterly 14,* 3, 363–382.

Law, J., Barnett, G. and Kot, A. (1999) 'Coding parent/child interaction as a clinical outcome: a research note.' *Child Language, Teaching and Therapy 1,* 261–275.

Locke, A., Ginsborg, J. and Peers, I. (2002) 'Development and disadvantage: implications for early years and beyond.' *International Journal of Language and Communication Disorders 37,* 1, 3–15.

Potter, C.A. (2005) *Sure Start Hinton: Quality of Play Reassessed.* Unpublished report.

Siraj-Blatchford, I., Sylva, K., Muttock, S., Gilden, R. and Bell, D. (2002) *Researching Effective Pedagogy in the Early Years.* Norwich: DfES.

Snow, C.E. (1991) 'The theoretical basis for relationships between language and literacy development.' *Journal of Research in Childhood Education 6,* 5–10.

Snow, C.E. and Paez, M. M. (2004) 'The Head Start classroom as an oral language environment: What should performance standards be?' In E. Zigler and S. J. Styfco (eds) *The Head Start Debates.* Baltimore, MD: Paul Brookes.

Ward, S. (1999) 'An investigation into the effectiveness of an early intervention method for delayed language development in young children.' *International Journal of Language and Communication Disorders 34,* 3, 243–264.

Wells, G. (1985) *Language Development in the Pre-school Years.* Cambridge: Cambridge University Press.

Chapter 7

A Perinatal Mental Health Project

Pauline Hall and Marjorie Finnigan

Postnatal (or postpartum) depression is generally estimated to affect around 10 to 15 per cent of women (O'Hara and Swain 1996; Rutter 1989). Since the last census (Office for National Statistics 2007) recorded approximately 695,500 births in the UK in 2003, postnatal depression represents a significant healthcare issue. The adverse effect of postnatal depression on infant outcomes is well documented. Research has shown that children of depressed mothers show poorer cognitive development (e.g. Lyons-Ruth, Connell and Grunebaum 1990), poorer emotional development (e.g. Murray 1992) and an increase in behavioural problems (e.g. Hubbs-Tait *et al.* 1996). Postnatal depression, therefore, gives rise to many adverse consequences for both mother and child. Adverse effects, however, also impact upon immediate family systems, as well as wider systems of social and healthcare networks. For example, women with depression receive proportionately more home visits from health visitors (Williams, Argent and Chalmers 1981), and the children of depressed mothers are taken to their general practitioner (GP) more often, receive more medication for minor childhood illness, and are more frequently admitted to hospital (Wolkind 1985).

The average cost of community care provided for women suffering from postnatal depression is significantly greater than that provided for women without the disorder. The economic cost of postnatal depression in terms of increased health and social care has been estimated at over £35 million in Britain per year (Civic and Holt 2000). Such a figure is likely to be an underestimate as their study only researched service use until the child was 18 months old. Effects of postnatal depression are likely to be longer lasting on both mother and child. In addition, other costs, such as travel and childcare, lost productivity and intangible costs (e.g. fear, pain and suffering), were not included (Petrou *et al.* 2002).

In contrast to postnatal depression, the study of depression during pregnancy has been relatively neglected. The Diagnostic and Statistical Manual (American Psychiatric Association 2000), used by psychiatrists to diagnose mental disorders, does not include a distinct category for antenatal depression.

Clinically, symptoms of depression in the antenatal period are similar to depressive symptoms in general, and include low mood, lack of energy, loss of enjoyment and feelings of guilt. Depression in the postnatal period is recognised as a separate condition from depression at other times in a woman's life, and routine screening is offered to most women in the UK at six to eight weeks postpartum. However, the need for formal recognition of antenatal depression may be equally important, as Evans *et al.* (2001) found depression scores were higher at 32 weeks of pregnancy than at eight weeks postpartum: 13.5 per cent of their sample (n=14,541) scored above threshold for depression at 32 weeks of pregnancy.

During pregnancy, women and healthcare professionals are often apprehensive about using medication to treat depression, even when indicated, for fear of harming the foetus. However, untreated depressed mood during pregnancy has been associated with poor attendance at antenatal clinics, substance misuse, low birth weight and preterm delivery. Furthermore, the biggest single predictor of postnatal depression is consistently found to be antenatal depression (Beck 1996; O'Hara and Swain 1996).

The imperative need to address maternal mental health issues was highlighted following the findings of the 'Confidential Enquiry into Maternal and Child Health' (CEMACH). The last two CEMACH reports published by the Royal College of Obstetricians and Gynaecologists (RCOG 2001, 2004), which examined UK maternal deaths within the periods 1997–1999 and 2000–2002, both concluded that psychiatric causes are the leading cause of death for mothers in the perinatal period (from conception up to one year post-delivery). The reports further revealed that mental illness leading to suicide was a major factor in a minimum of 10 per cent of maternal deaths. The means of suicide was most commonly violent and, as such, differs from the most common means in non-postnatal women (overdose). In response to the consistent finding that suicide is the most frequent cause of death in mothers during the first year after delivery, recommendations included access for women to specialist perinatal mental health teams.

The CEMACH reports also recognised that the most effective way of protecting mother and child is to detect the illness. Recommendations included that midwives ask women at their initial visit about previous psychiatric illness, that professionals offer shared multidisciplinary care when there are complex social issues, including mental health problems, and that there is the development of a management plan which involves the midwife, obstetrician, GP, psychiatrist and family. However, the report also states that these strategies should be put in place only after midwives have received appropriate training and updates on mental health detection and services.

Service initiative: the Perinatal Project

The Perinatal Project is a local partnership between Salford Sure Start, Bolton, Salford and Trafford NHS Mental Health Trust and Salford Royal Hospital NHS Trust. The service comprises a specialist perinatal mental health team working with antenatal and postnatal women who are suffering from, or at risk of, depression. As well as direct clinical work, the service offers consultation and training to other staff members. This peripatetic service therefore meets the recommendations of the CEMACH reports as well as other government legislation, such as *The National Service Framework (NSF) for Children, Young People and Maternity Services* (Department of Health 2004) and the current guidelines for treatment of antenatal and postnatal mental health (National Collaborating Centre for Mental Health 2006).

The Perinatal Project began in 2003 in the Sure Start areas of Salford. Set up by a midwifery lead, together with a steering group, the service was funded by Sure Start monies. Rates of postpartum depression in the Sure Start areas of Salford were found to be as high as 47 per cent, which is nearly four times the national average of 13 per cent (O'Hara and Swain 1996). The Perinatal Project was pioneered to address specific Sure Start objectives, including improving the health and emotional well-being of children, and improving the psychological well-being of women (Lythgoe 2006).

Women may be referred to the Perinatal Project via their GP, midwife or health visitor. Guidelines regarding referral pathways to the Perinatal Project are outlined in Figure 7.1a and 7.1b.

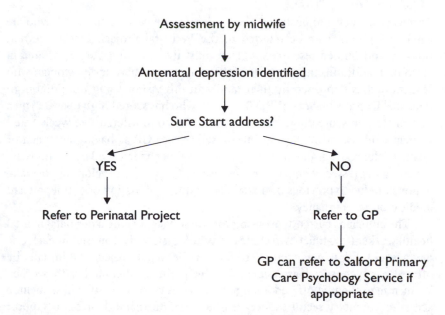

Figure 7.1a Salford guidelines for the management of antenatal depression

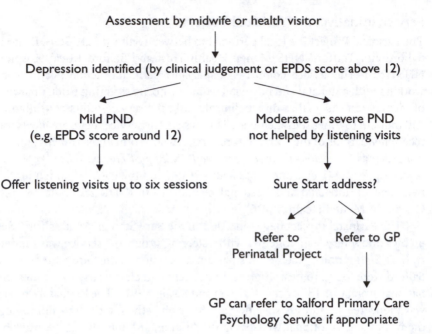

Figure 7.1b Salford guidelines for the management of postnatal depression (PND)

Eligibility for the service

Antenatal women and postnatal women (up to one year postpartum), who are aged 16 or over, may be referred to the Perinatal Project. Due to current funding and limited resources, women must live within a Sure Start area in Salford. In addition, any one of the following criteria may apply: woman who is identified as depressed by their family health visitor using the Edinburgh Postnatal Depression Scale (EPDS); woman who has scored high (over 12) on a first EPDS and scored high on a second EPDS administered two weeks later; woman who has been seen and diagnosed by her GP as having antenatal or postnatal depression; antenatal woman who has been identified by her midwife as feeling depressed; woman identified as at high risk for developing postnatal depression due to previous postnatal depression or cessation of antidepressant medication in pregnancy.

The clinicians currently working for the service include a perinatal mental health worker (full-time), two clinical psychologists and a counsellor (each one day a week). Eligible women referred to the Perinatal Project will initially be offered a psychosocial assessment by the perinatal mental health worker. Women may then be offered a range of services or treatments. These include access to voluntary sector services (e.g. Relate), postnatal depression support groups, or a range of psychological therapies delivered by the Perinatal

Project clinical psychologists or counsellor. Possible pathways are illustrated in Figure 7.2.

The Perinatal Project aims to offer a psychosocial assessment within six weeks of referral. As the service is not resourced to act as an emergency service, referrers are advised that if depression is severe then referral should be made more appropriately to a community mental health team or, if risk is immediate, to an accident and emergency crisis team. In the event of any child protection concerns, referrers are advised to contact social services. Assessment and treatment facilities currently directly available within the Perinatal Project are shown in Figure 7.3.

In addition to direct client assessment and intervention, the Perinatal Project offers training for all midwives and health visitors in Salford. A consultancy service for professionals working with Sure Start and non-Sure Start women offers advice on other services and means of referral. Staff using the consultancy service have represented a range of agencies, including primary care trusts (PCTs), general practice surgeries and community mental health teams.

Delivery of perinatal depression training

As part of the service delivered by the Perinatal Project clinical team, teaching days on perinatal depression have been offered to relevant staff. Training was offered to all health visitors, all community midwives and many of the hospital-based midwives, such as the drug liaison midwife, the neonatal outreach sisters and neonatal intensive care unit staff. In total, ten teaching days were conducted from July to September 2005. During this time, training was delivered to 32 midwives, 57 health visitors and six others (assistant psychologists, staff nurses and the Perinatal Project administrator).

The content of the day included an introduction and overview, understanding antenatal and postnatal depression, risk assessment and management, confidential inquiry findings (what to ask, action to take), research in perinatal depression, counselling skills, and when and where to refer. The training also included guidance on how to complete the EPDS, both with antenatal and postnatal women. This is a well validated screening tool (Cox, Holden and Sagovsky 1987) to identify women who may be suffering from postnatal depression. Although it is not usually recommended as a screening tool in the antenatal period, it was considered useful and appropriate to introduce this during pregnancy to help raise awareness of depression in the perinatal period. Training was also delivered to nursery nurses employed by Salford PCT and all Sure Start workers. This training aimed to raise awareness of perinatal depression, its debilitating effects, and who to contact in the case of concerns that a woman may be depressed. In total, the Perinatal Project team has trained over 130 staff, including those groups already mentioned and others who may have contact with women who could access the service (e.g. the Jewish Federation).

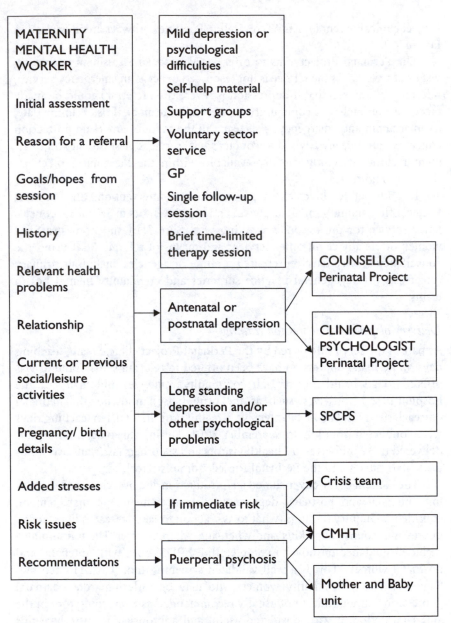

Key:

SPCPS: Salford Primary Care Psychology Service

Crisis Team: A&E Liaison Crisis Team

CMHT: Community Mental Health Team

Figure 7.2 Perinatal Project guidelines for assessment of psychological problems

1. Psychosocial assessment by the perinatal mental health worker within six weeks of referral.

2. Two postnatal depression support groups.

3. Individual counselling.

4. Individual psychological therapy.

5. Perinatal depression training for all midwives, health visitors and other relevant staff.

6. Multi-agency liaison, including relevant presentations.

7. A consultancy service for professionals working with antenatal and postnatal women.

Figure 7.3 The range of current services within the Perinatal Project

Training was arranged at local NHS and Sure Start venues which did not incur any charge. The training was delivered by one of the perinatal team psychologists and the perinatal mental health worker with contributions from the other team members. Due to the specialist knowledge and experience of the team, it was not felt necessary to employ external speakers. The teaching style involved didactic presentations, small group work and interactive discussions. Opportunities for questions and clarification were given throughout. Attendees were each given a pack containing handouts of the presentation slides in addition to other relevant information (e.g. copies of the scales, referral contact names and details). Packs were photocopied and compiled by an assistant psychologist. The training programme therefore achieved a high standard of delivery on a low and cost-effective budget.

Evaluation of perinatal depression training

The perinatal depression training has received very positive feedback. The feedback data are summarised in Table 7.1. Attendees were asked to rate each item on a scale of nought to ten, where nought indicates poor quality and ten excellent quality.

Attendees were also asked on the feedback form to note any suggestions for improvement. Six attendees noted that the venue could be improved as some of the rooms which were used were quite small. Two attendees suggested that involvement of GPs in such training sessions would be useful. Other comments reflected positive feedback, as well as suggestions for improvement: 'Interesting, relevant and enjoyable. Need regular updates'; 'This has been a very good, informative session which will be useful for everyday working and added greatly to knowledge base'; 'Very little needed to improve. Perhaps more about clinical "tips" on how to manage antenatal depression as this is fairly neglected

Table 7.1 Perinatal depression training feedback

	Mean	Median	Mode
Session content			
Background information	9.09	9.00	10
Coverage of approach	9.22	9.00	10
Relevance to pratice	9.47	10.00	10
Level of enjoyment	9.17	9.00	10
Teaching style			
Quality of presentation slides	9.36	10.00	10
Structure of session	9.19	9.00	10
Opportunity for questions	9.58	10.00	10
Clarity of lecturing style	9.40	10.00	10

area'; 'Great to get a better understanding and now feel more positive about dealing with this problem'.

Evaluation of clinical work

Rigorous evaluation has been an important consideration in the development of the service. All women who were referred to the project completed an EPDS to measure severity of depression. An initial aim was to send women an anonymous feedback questionnaire asking about the usefulness of the service, how they benefited from the service and any improvements that could be made. There was an opportunity for women to give their name and contact details if they were prepared to be interviewed by a trained member of the Sure Start evaluation team from Salford University. This would involve a semistructured interview about their use of the service and how effective it had been for them. However, response rates from postal questionnaires are known to be low (Fife-Schaw 2000) and unfortunately very few women returned completed forms. Thus reconsideration of the evaluation strategy was necessary. The option of asking women to complete the feedback questionnaire during the final therapy session was considered, but it was felt that this might give rise to biased favourable responses if women did not feel comfortable completing this whilst the therapist was present. Verbal anecdotal evidence from women who used the service was collected more successfully. Comments included: 'I wish it had been available with my first child'; 'It made me realise I was not mad'; 'I'm finding it really useful to talk to someone who understands how I feel', and 'My anxiety has really improved, I feel normal again'.

In addition, anecdotal evidence from referrers was positive. Their comments included: 'Great for immediate referral for women in need' (midwife); 'It is really important that mums are able to get quick and easy access to such a valuable service' (health visitor); 'It is great to have such a service so women are seen quickly and interventions commenced. I wish we had it for all our patients, not just those in the Sure Start area' (GP).

In order to provide more rigorous evaluative data, however, it was decided to ask all the women who received therapy to complete a set of measures at the start and completion of therapy. A comparison of the pre- and post-therapy scores would thus demonstrate any improvements in their mental health. The measures used are the EPDS (Cox *et al.* 1987), Postnatal Negative Thoughts Questionnaire (Hall and Papageorgiou 2005), Self-Evaluation Questionnaire (Spielberger 1989), Robson Self-Concept Questionnaire (Robson 1989) and the General Health Questionnaire (Goldberg 1972). All measures have been well validated and are suitable for use with a perinatal population. In order to promote completion of the post-therapy measures with honest responses, the women are offered a home visit by an assistant psychologist to complete the assessments.

Proposals for further development

The Perinatal Project has been well received and supported by clients and referrers to date. Sympathetic to the needs of pregnant or new mothers and their families, the Perinatal Project offers women priority access to specialised psychological assessment and treatment to ameliorate mental distress in the perinatal period. Expansion of the service is hoped for in order to meet the identified need of the local community.

Preliminary work to develop a ten-session postnatal depression treatment group, based upon the Webster-Stratton 'Parent Survival Course', has also been undertaken. Research studies have shown that Webster-Stratton groups are efficacious in not only improving child behaviour problems but also in decreasing parental depression (Webster-Stratton 1990; White, Agnew and Verduyn 2002). Webster-Stratton groups, however, are currently aimed at parents of children from ages three to eight. Clearly, those suffering postnatal depression suffer adverse effects when their children are much younger. A protocol has therefore been developed which specifically addresses the needs of depressed parents of babies up to one year of age. The content has been written as a joint initiative between child and adult psychology services and, as such, offers a unique opportunity for working across service boundaries for the benefit of children and parents. Information leaflets for parents and referrers have also been developed and resources are already available (e.g. video camera). In addition, all clinical staff on the Perinatal Project have been trained in Webster-Stratton parenting approaches. Although the Perinatal Project currently offers two postnatal depression support groups, the new proposed group will serve as an important addition: it will be closed, didactic and experiential to deliver psychological therapy specifically. The group will also offer a fantastic treatment option, in addition to the individual work currently conducted by the therapists, as more women can be seen at any one time, and the benefits of peer support in group work for the treatment of postnatal depression may be promoted.

In addition to running a rolling programme of the perinatal teaching day for new staff members, it is proposed that a second half-day of training will offer an opportunity for staff to reflect on day one, seek clarification on any issues previously discussed and review how practice has changed as a result of the training. In addition, day two content will include teaching on important aspects not covered in day one due to time limitations. The proposed agenda includes introduction and recap, reflective practice and questions, overview of treatments for antenatal and postnatal depression, medication, cognitive behaviour therapy and children's issues.

The role for Children's Centres

Sure Start aims to improve outcomes and opportunities for children, parents and communities by improving the health and emotional development of young children. The Department for Education and Skills (now the Department for Children, Schools and Families) Standards website states the aims of the Children's Centres programme as being to have 'broad and lasting impact on children, their parents and the wider community' (Every Child Matters 2007), and that one of the goals of the Children's Centres will be to contribute towards the government's commitment to the best start in life for every child.

Clearly, from the evidence available, it will not be possible to achieve these outcomes without reference to maternal mental health. Children's Centres face a very complex and difficult task in attempting to give children the best start in life when this is influenced by so many variables. Addressing a child's physical and mental well-being and educational status will undoubtedly contribute towards reaching this goal, but if maternal mental health is not considered in the process, any gains made in these other areas are likely to be reduced by the effect of the mother's poor mental health. Improved maternal mental health, achieved through services such as the Perinatal Project, can have a positive impact on the health and safety of children. Furthermore, the members of the Perinatal Project are all trained in the Webster-Stratton approach to parenting and have child-development training. This enables a more holistic and integrated approach to the problems that families may present with, and reduces the necessity for referrals across to child psychology services. As well as providing a more streamlined service, this helps to avoid some of the difficulties which might be encountered when numerous professionals from different services become involved in complex family systems.

The Perinatal Project contributes to giving children the best start in life by reducing the barrier which perinatal depression can impose on a mother's ability to bond with and care for her children to the best of her ability. Depressed women easily become trapped in patterns of negative thinking which lead to thoughts of being a bad mother and this, in turn, lowers their mood further, thus creating a vicious cycle. The effect of perinatal depression on the mother–child relationship, and its effect on the child's cognitive, emotional and behavioural development, will not be ameliorated by any amount of input to the child's health whilst the child remains in an environment where the mother's health issues are not addressed. Therefore, in order to meet the standards set out in *The National Service Framework for Children, Young People and Maternity Services* (Department of Health 2004), and for the benefit of women, children and families, it is imperative that priority access to specialised mental health services is offered to all mothers in the perinatal period.

Due to resource limitations and a high demand to meet client need, expansion of the Perinatal Project to operate city-wide will require additional funding of staff time in order to maintain and develop the benefits already achieved. Applications for continued and extra funding are therefore currently being made. It is very much hoped this will be successful in order to continue to deliver a high quality perinatal mental health service to antenatal and postnatal women in Salford.

Implications for Children's Centres

- The adverse effects of perinatal depression on infant development are well established and include poor cognitive, emotional and behavioural development.

- In order to meet Children's Centre aims, and recommendations from government directives, including the children's National Service Framework, it is imperative that services address maternal mental health.

- The Salford Perinatal Project offers a model of good practice for the development and delivery of a service to meet the mental health needs of a perinatal population for the benefit of women, children and families.

Acknowledgements

Thank you to Jeanne Lythgoe for all her hard work and initiation of the project. We would also like to acknowledge our other team members, Suzanne Glendenning and Cathy Worthy, and express our thanks and appreciation to the women of Salford who have participated in our service.

References

American Psychiatric Association (2000) *Diagnostic and Statistical Manual of Mental Disorders* (4th edition, text revised). Washington, DC: American Psychiatric Press.

Beck, C.T. (1996) 'A meta-analysis of predictors of postpartum depression.' *Nursing Research 45*, 5, 297–303.

Civic, D. and Holt, V.L. (2000) 'Maternal depressive symptoms and child behaviour problems in a nationally representative normal birthweight sample.' *Maternal and Child Health Journal 4*, 4, 215–221.

Cox, J.L., Holden, J.M. and Sagovsky, R. (1987) 'Detection of postnatal depression: development of the 10-item Edinburgh Postnatal Depression Scale.' *British Journal of Psychiatry 150*, 6, 782–786.

Department of Health (2004) *The National Service Framework for Children, Young People and Maternity Services*. London: DoH.

Evans, J., Heron, J., Francomb, H., Oke, S. and Golding, J. (2001) 'Cohort study of depressed mood during pregnancy and after childbirth.' *British Medical Journal 323*, 7307, 257–260.

Every Child Matters (2007) 'Sure Start children's centres.' www.everychildmatters.gov.uk/earlyyears/surestart/centres, accessed on 17 October 2007.

Fife-Schaw, C. (2000) 'Surveys and sampling bias.' In G. Brakell, S. Hammond and C. Fife-Schaw (eds) *Research Methods and Psychology* (2nd edition). London: Sage.

Goldberg, D.P. (1972) *The Detection of Psychiatric Illness by Questionnaire*. London: Oxford University Press.

Hall, P.L. and Papageorgiou, C. (2005) 'Negative thoughts after childbirth: development and preliminary validation of a self-report scale.' *Depression and Anxiety 22*, 3, 121–129.

Hubbs-Tait, L., Hughes, K.P., Culp, A.M., Osofsky, J.D., Hann, D.M., Eberhart-Wright, A. and Ware, L.M. (1996) 'Children of adolescent mothers: attachment representation, maternal depression and later behaviour problems.' *American Journal of Orthopsychiatry 66*, 3, 416–426.

Lyons-Ruth, K., Connell, D.B. and Grunebaum, H.U. (1990) 'Infants at social risk: maternal depression and family support services as mediators of infant development and security of attachment.' *Child Development 61*, 1, 85–98.

Lythgoe, J. (2006) *Sure Start Midwifery Evaluation 2003–2006*. Salford: Sure Start Midwifery Project.

Murray, L. (1992) 'The impact of postnatal depression on infant development.' *Journal of Child Psychology and Psychiatry 33*, 3, 543–561.

National Collaborating Centre for Mental Health (2006) *Antenatal and Postnatal Mental Health: Clinical Management and Service Guidelines. NICE guideline*. Draft for Consultation.

Office for National Statistics (2007) www.statistics.gov.uk, accessed on 5 January 2007.

O'Hara, M.W. and Swain, A.M. (1996) 'Rates and risks of postpartum depression: a meta-analysis.' *International Review of Psychiatry 8*, 4, 37–54.

Petrou, S., Cooper, P., Murray, L. and Davidson, L.L. (2002) 'Economic costs of postnatal depression in a high-risk British cohort.' *British Journal of Psychiatry 181*, 6, 505–512.

Robson, P. (1989) 'Development of a new self report questionnaire to measure self-esteem.' *Psychological Medicine 19*, 2, 513–518.

Royal College of Obstetricians and Gynaecologists (2001) *Why Mothers Die 1997–1999: the Fifth Report of the Confidential Enquiries into Maternal and Child Health in the United Kingdom*. London: RCOG.

Royal College of Obstetricians and Gynaecologists (2004) *Why Mothers Die 2000–2002: the Sixth Report of the Confidential Enquiries into Maternal and Child Health in the United Kingdom*. London: RCOG.

Rutter, M. (1989) 'Psychiatric disorder in parents as a risk factor for children.' In D. Schaffer, I. Philips and N.B. Enger (eds) *Prevention of Mental Disorder, Alcohol and Other Drug Use in Children and Adolescents*. Rockville, MD: Office of Substance Abuse.

Spielberger, C.D. (1989) *State-Trait Anxiety Inventory: a Comprehensive Bibliography*. Palo Alto, CA: Consulting Psychologists Press.

Webster-Stratton, C. (1990) 'Long-term follow-up of families with young conduct-problem children: from pre-school to grade school.' *Journal of Clinical Child Psychology 19*, 2, 144–149.

White, C., Agnew, J. and Verduyn, C. (2002). 'The Little Hulton Project: a pilot child clinical psychology service for pre-school children and their families.' *Child and Adolescent Mental Health 7*, 1, 10–15.

Williams, P.R., Argent, E.M.H. and Chalmers, C. (1981) 'A study of an urban health centre: factors influencing contact with mothers and their babies.' *Child Care, Health and Development 7*, 5, 255–266.

Wolkind, S. (1985) 'Mothers' depression and their children's attendance at medical facilities.' *Journal of Psychosomatic Research 29*, 6, 579–582.

Part 2

Partnership Working

Chapter 8

Introduction to Partnership Working

Paul Leighton

Sure Start is a multidisciplinary programme of social and healthcare services and interventions targeted to young families in areas of social and economic disadvantage. It is an initiative that rests in the notion that the multiple and interconnected symptoms of social exclusion (poor health, poor educational attainment, limited aspiration, family breakdown and community decline, to name but a few) call for joined-up solutions which span traditional disciplinary and service delivery demarcations. Geographic targeting and broad-based objectives, such as improving health, improving learning, strengthening families and communities and improving social and emotional development, further challenge traditional lines of service delivery and have encouraged Sure Start Local Programmes (SSLPs) to think holistically (and locally) about social issues. Multi-agency and partnership working have consequently been signifi-cant characteristics of SSLPs. Local programme teams are, in the main, multidisciplinary (often with strong connections to local statutory service pro-viders), and programmes have worked with and alongside statutory service providers, community and voluntary groups, the private sector and local parents to address complex social issues and to respond to distinctive local circumstances.

Such partnership working is often presented unproblematically as auto-matically beneficial if the purely *technical* issues of communication and substantive focus can be established. For example, Myers, Barnes and Brodie (2004) recognise that, amongst SSLPs, partnership working is perceived to be a necessary and productive way of shaping and delivering services. However, partnership working can often be a site of tension and difficulty, worthy of more considered attention.

Tunstill *et al.* (2005) recognise two broad forms of partnership working that can be found, to a greater or lesser degree, in all SSLPs: *a partnership board* approach and *a partnership way of working*. The former demonstrates a concern for *the involvement of parents in the design, management and delivery of services*, whilst the latter is about service providers *joining up for Sure Start*, coordinating their activities and investment (Eisenstadt 2002). The chapters presented here will consider both these forms of partnership working.

First of all, Wigfall *et al.* in Chapter 9 and Graham in Chapter 10 explore partnership with local parents in the operation of SSLPs. One of the key and most distinctive features of the Sure Start agenda was a commitment to community consultation and involving local parents in shaping and organising services: '[government] Ministers have defined the problem and set the framework. Local people are designing and delivering the solution' (Eisenstadt 2002, p.4). Parental involvement in the creation of SSLPs and then in their operation, through participation in management boards, task groups and parent forums, was intended to ensure local flavour to provision, a responsiveness to local circumstances and, most of all, services and activities that parents would want and support. However, the chapters presented here demonstrate that this apparently uncomplicated agenda is in fact complex and influenced by a range of local and broader features. Graham (Chapter 10) considers *parental self-esteem, the status of the child and professional autonomy* in likening the professional/parent relationship within Sure Start to that between parent and child. Wigfall *et al.* (Chapter 9) explore a continuum of parental involvement which ranges from simple awareness of Sure Start to being active decision-makers and service leaders.

In both these chapters a concern for status, power and role inequalities is evident as the authors recognise the importance of a 'bottom-up' approach to parental involvement and to parent partnership. Wigfall *et al.* recognise the importance of a non-hierarchical and overlapping model of parental involvement which validates and supports Sure Start participation in all forms. Graham calls for sensitivity and flexibility on the part of professionals in their dealing with Sure Start parents in an attempt to renegotiate an otherwise unequal relationship. Both chapters recognise that partnerships with parents occur at many levels within SSLPs, from sharing play activities with children to the level of strategic management. Both also recognise the important role that staff play in facilitating and maintaining these relationships.

Griffin and Carpenter (Chapter 11) and Edgley (Chapter 12) consider partnership working and SSLPs' relationship with other service providers. This is an important aspect of Sure Start's innovative agenda which is intended to prevent the replication of provision and ensure that issues are tackled in a holistic and concerted fashion. From the outset local programmes were designed 'to build upon services that already exist in the area', whilst 'all [local] services are expected to contribute to achieving Sure Start's objectives' (Eisenstadt 2002). Therefore, one of the key challenges for many local programmes was to create an environment where multi-agency working and active local partnerships could flourish. These two chapters presented here consider some of the complexities of this issue.

Griffin and Carpenter explore the relationship between Sure Start and social service departments in eight local programmes in the north-east. Utilising two complementary models of partnership and involvement they recognise a complex set of circumstances which are influenced both by national policy developments and by local experiences and expectations. In a similar vein Edgley suggests that Sure Start's significance lies less in creating a new ethos of partnership working and more in offering the funding to support existing *local* collaborations and professionals who are already sensitive to the benefits of integrated, multi-professional working. Both these chapters flag the complex set of relationships that exist between local circumstances (e.g. professionals who already know each other), broader service delivery developments (e.g. the role and remit of social service departments) and the stipulations and requirements of the Sure Start agenda (i.e. substantively and geographically targeted) in establishing effective local partnerships. Sure Start can be seen both to have facilitated partnership working, in the funding and impetus that it offers to this type of approach, and to constrain partnership working where geographic boundaries and substantive interests do not match and where awareness of different models of service delivery is poor.

With a transition to a Children's Centre model of service delivery it might be suggested that the challenge of partnership working not only remains but is significantly enhanced. The *core offer* of services that each centre must provide stipulates an integrated approach which brings together *education, childcare, health and family support* (Department for Education and Skills 2003). This calls for the involvement of the *private, voluntary and independent sectors* (Department for Education and Skills 2006), although it may be that it is more restricted funding, and different models of service management, that truly create the strongest motivation for greater partnership working. The removal of (generous) ring-fenced Sure Start funding ensures that local authorities, who assume responsibility for managing Children's Centres, have to work more directly with a range of partner agencies to achieve multidimensional service delivery. The lessons that can be taken from SSLP experiences of partnership working perhaps become more, rather than less, significant as Children's Centres become established.

The importance of parental involvement is, however, perhaps less clear-cut. Reduced funding and less autonomy for individual Children's Centres suggest that the potential for parental involvement in decision-making processes might be significantly reduced; yet this is an area where SSLPs were perceived to be a real success, and to have had a significant impact upon both individuals and communities (Glass 2005). So whilst Children's Centres might not be *owned* by parents in the same way that SSLPs were, the lessons that can be taken from SSLPs about how to engage with and involve parents should not be lost, and should be built into the way that Children's Centres grow and are developed.

References

Department for Education and Skills (2003) *Sure Start Guidance, 2004–2006: Section II Delivery Guidance.* Nottingham: DfES Publications.

Department for Education and Skills (2006) *Sure Start Children's Centres Planning and Performance Management Guidance.* Nottingham: DfES Publications.

Eisenstadt, N. (2002) 'Sure Start: key principles and ethos.' *Child: Care, Health and Development 28*, 1, 3–4.

Glass, N. (2005) 'Surely some mistake.' *The Guardian (education section)*, 5 January 2005.

Myers, P., Barnes, J. and Brodie, I. (2004) *Partnership Working in Sure Start Local Programmes – Synthesis of Early Findings from Local Programme Evaluations.* London: Sure Start Unit.

Tunstill, J., Meadows, P., Allnock, D., Akhurst, S., Chrysanthou, J., Garbers, C., Morley, A. and van de Velde, T. (2005) *Implementing Sure Start Local Programmes: An In-depth Study.* Nottingham: DfES Publications.

Chapter 9

Parental Involvement: Engagement with the Development of Services

Valerie Wigfall, Janet Boddy and Susan McQuail

One of the most significant features of the Sure Start initiative has been its commitment to the involvement of parents, both as users and in the governance of the programmes. Programmes have been able to respond to locally identified needs, and have been led and delivered through a partnership board of local stakeholders which has included parents. Thus parents have had a strong voice in determining what services are to be developed. Sure Start's vision has aimed to overcome barriers that have traditionally prevented or discouraged certain groups from accessing or using the services on offer (Kempson and Whyley 1999; Sanderson 2002) and to promote the widest possible engagement in the whole range of Sure Start activities.

This chapter explores what the concept of parent involvement means in practice, and describes its varied translation across six Sure Start Local Programmes (SSLPs) that participated in an evaluation of parent involvement undertaken for a London borough.

Background to the study

Like many local authorities in London, the borough that sponsored this study is characterised by contrasts. Geographically it is one of the smallest, but also one of the most densely populated local authorities in the country, with a total of nearly 200,000 residents (Office for National Statistics 2001). Socio-economically, the population is mixed, with a high proportion of workers in professional and managerial occupations, but overall the area ranks as one of the most deprived in the country, according to the Office of the Deputy Prime Minister's (ODPM) Indices of Deprivation 2004 (ODPM 2004). One in ten households has children aged 0–4 years.

At the time of the evaluation, the borough hosted six SSLPs, all of which were included in the evaluation. They provided services to families of children up to the age of four in areas covering just over half the borough. All the programmes were situated within socioeconomically deprived wards, and all served ethnically diverse populations. At the time of the evaluation, each SSLP had a budget in the region of £0.78 million. The six programmes were at varying stages in the process of becoming Children's Centres, reflecting their different ages and histories.

The evaluation

The evaluation focused on two complementary facets of the local programmes' work: intensive family support and parent involvement (Boddy, McQuail and Wigfall 2005). This chapter addresses primarily the latter, while acknowledging that Sure Start family support services can provide an important route into parent involvement for some families. The study was commissioned to inform strategic developments for Early Years children's services within the authority, particularly with regard to the Children's Centre Programme and mainstreaming of services for young children and their families. The specific objectives of the parent involvement element of the study were:

- to determine how parents become involved with SSLPs, including involvement in local programme activities, parents' forums and board meetings.
- to develop an understanding of what involvement means for parents and their children.

Methodology

In addition to a review of relevant documentation and visits by the research team to parent forum meetings in each programme, the following interviews were carried out:

- four interviews with Sure Start staff in each of the six local programmes, including programme managers, family support workers and parent involvement workers (total 24 workers interviewed)
- 12 telephone interviews with representatives of relevant linked external agencies from health, social services, early years and the voluntary sector
- 60 telephone interviews (up to ten per programme) of parents (including six fathers) who had used services in May 2005. These parents were randomly selected from membership lists held by the local programmes, with consecutive replacement sampling to ensure representation of members of minority ethnic groups, parents of children with special needs, parent forum members, and fathers. The socioeconomic status of the respondents reflected that in the

borough as a whole, including English, 16 different languages were spoken in the home.

What is parent involvement?

Responding to this question, a programme manager gave the following answer:

> Parent involvement is involving them in activities…the purpose of parent involvement is finding out what parents want, and making sure they get what they want, not what providers think they want.

Yet this comment explains only part of the continuum of participation identified when we started to examine the different ways in which parents became involved in the SSLPs. Operating at different levels, this continuum reflects in some ways the classic 'ladder of participation' first developed by Sherry Arnstein in the USA in the 1960s to model the ways in which people can influence public programmes (Arnstein 1969) and adapted subsequently by Hart in this country to describe young people's participation (Hart 1992). However, both of these models are hierarchical, relating very much to power and governance, and thus did not wholly reflect the model of developing involvement that we observed. Rather more appropriate in the present context is Tunstill and colleagues' account of a continuum of access to services (2005a) in relation to the implementation of Sure Start, whereby the links which local programmes make with local families may extend across a range of possibilities which are not mutually exclusive, from initial contact via leafleting or outreach, through various degrees of access, up to autonomous take-up of services other than those provided by Sure Start.

In much the same way, we could see from our research that involvement, like access to services, may include a variety of different levels of participation. At one end, it might refer simply to engagement of families who are potentially 'hard-to-reach', making sure they know what services are available and encouraging them to use them. Moving on from there, taking up services is in itself a way of getting involved as a user. At another level, so too is participation through consultation, allowing users to 'have a say' to ensure that what is provided is what people want. Finally, parents from local communities might develop capacity to run their own services, by serving actively on a forum or programme board, whereby involvement becomes more instrumental in shaping and developing services. Thus, the notion of a continuum (Figure 9.1) effectively describes these different levels of involvement. Levels are non-hierarchical and overlapping: families might move back and forth along the continuum over time. They might become involved in Sure Start in one or more ways as they become informed or as they feel able or indeed wish. This model is inclusive, embracing involvement in both formal and informal ways, and reflects the 'bottom-up' community development perspective that the Sure

Start local programmes sought to establish. The challenge for them has been engaging parents in these various ways, and recognising the validity of each.

This broad interpretation of parent involvement sits within one of the key principles to which all Sure Start Local Programmes have been expected to work: promoting the participation of *all* local families in the design, management and delivery of the Sure Start programmes (Eisenstadt 2002).

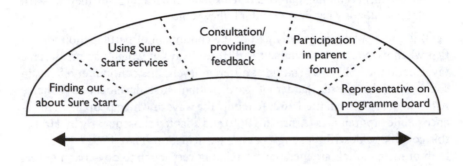

Figure 9.1 A continuum of involvement

The six SSLPs reflected different approaches to parent involvement in planning and organisation and the degree of emphasis placed upon it. Across the six programmes, all the Sure Start workers interviewed said that parent involvement was and would continue to be at the heart of service delivery. Most programmes had a dedicated parent involvement worker, although titles and roles varied. In addition to encouraging participation at the formal levels of parent forums and programme boards, responsibilities of these workers included publicity, outreach, consultation, development of volunteer activities, events organisation, and training. In one case, the parent involvement post was combined with a training and employment post; in another, with the post of outreach worker. Some programmes had recently employed link workers who spoke community languages to increase outreach to parents from ethnic minority groups. One parent involvement post was at a senior level, reflecting the importance placed on this role by the programme manager. This programme had the highest level of parent involvement of all the programmes studied.

What was clear was that a dedicated staff role appeared to strengthen the level of parent involvement, particularly in supporting parents to move along the continuum towards more active involvement in groups like the parent forum or the programme board. For example, in one programme, attendance of the parent forum dropped to zero in a two-month period when the parent involvement worker took a period of leave.

Three parent involvement workers were local parents (two were former Sure Start parents), which was said by managers to bring the 'bonus' of familiarity with the local area and residents. Formal qualifications varied. 'People skills' and common sense were generally thought more important than previous work experience, although being a parent, having an understanding of families and children, and experience in community development were all thought to be relevant.

Finding out about Sure Start and participation in activities

To varying degrees, all six programmes had engaged families living in diverse socioeconomic circumstances, and who reflected the ethnic composition of the neighbourhoods in which they were located.

The 60 parents interviewed were asked how they had heard about Sure Start. Publicity (mailshots, notices) played a key part in bringing in the parents defined by Tunstill *et al.* (2005a) as 'autonomous', that is, parents who readily take up services without prompting or support. However, health visitors and Sure Start workers were the most common route to finding out about Sure Start for parents from less socioeconomically advantaged backgrounds, and particularly for those who were receiving intensive family support services from the programmes. These findings indicated the importance of outreach in attracting families often classed as 'hard-to-reach', for whom written material might be less effective.

Like most Sure Start programmes, a wide range of activities was on offer in the six programmes studied, for both children and parents, for example stay and play, music and dance, baby massage, first aid, smoking cessation. Parents interviewed had tried on average four different types of activity. The most commonly used were stay and play (43/60), crèche facilities (25/60), and trips and outings (24/60). Only four parents said they had not found it easy to use Sure Start services. Most made positive comments about becoming involved. One parent described how she knew the staff team by name: 'I feel part of [Sure Start] and made to feel welcome'. Another had become involved after taking her child swimming: 'Once I got there I realised how easy it was. I had thought it would be difficult to manage changing with the baby in the buggy. If I'd realised I would have started sooner'. Over half (36/60) said support from a Sure Start worker had helped or encouraged them to get involved, for example a telephone invitation or an escort on the first visit.

There was no evidence of systematic problems preventing participation, but examples of individual experiences included practical difficulties transporting young children from a flat with no lift, lack of support in the group for a disabled child, language issues, or simply inconvenience in the timing of activities for working parents.

Giving feedback

Finding out what parents want is an essential part of a parent-led programme. Over half of the parent sample (36/60) had previously given some kind of feedback on Sure Start services, although percentages varied considerably between the six programmes, from 30 per cent to 90 per cent, and were generally lower for those for whom English was not the main language. Interviewees were also asked how they would prefer to give feedback. Most preferred direct methods – informal conversations with staff, telephone surveys, questionnaires at activities – and few suggested feeding back indirectly through a parent representative at a parents' forum. Few parents were aware of changes that had resulted from their feedback, suggesting that programmes could perhaps benefit from wider dissemination of feedback. As one parent remarked, 'It doesn't matter which way [I give feedback] as long as I feel listened to.'

Parent forum

All six programmes had a group known as the parent forum, or similar, which met regularly. The parent forum was open to all parents; formal membership was not a requirement. There were no terms of office, and parents could attend whenever they wished. Parents across the whole range of Sure Start activities were encouraged to attend the meetings. Most programmes tended to have a core group of parents who came regularly, but one programme, notably when there was no parent involvement worker, had struggled to maintain even a core group.

Managers suggested that the function of the parent forum was bringing parents and staff together in a relaxed setting to promote feedback and generate ideas for shaping services. To this extent, the forum was in some respects the cornerstone of parent involvement. Parents could come and speak up, or simply listen, without getting involved in management issues. One local parent described the role of the forum as 'looking at what we want, as well as what the children want, and what everyone else wants that's around, so that everyone can come and join in, which is really good'. The forum could be a place where parents came to 'moan' or 'complain' or a place for 'constructive criticism'. A more general function was to provide a communication channel between the parents' forum and the more formal programme board (see below).

Sure Start workers played a key role in encouraging parent involvement in the parents' forum, trying to achieve a good cross section of parents, and also in facilitating the forum's work. Certain parent groups had clearly been harder to reach, such as fathers, working parents, parents of children with special needs, and parents from black and minority ethnic groups, particularly those for whom English was not the first language. With this last group, link workers who spoke community languages were said to have made a difference. They occasionally accompanied parents to forum meetings, a useful role in overcoming parents' negative perceptions of the group. One parent described how she had been put off at her first visit: 'I feel they all know each other, I looked in once and then walked out'. Yet she suggested that had a member of staff accompanied her she might have felt differently.

Awareness of the forums was quite low among parents taking part in telephone interviews. At least four out of ten parents in each of the six local programmes did not know what the forum was or had never attended one, and few parents who were not already involved expressed an interest in actively participating, although just over half of these said they might like to attend occasionally. Inconvenience and the commitment required were the most commonly mentioned barriers to regular involvement.

For those parents who had taken part in forum meetings, the importance of the forum went beyond gathering parental views. One mother described how she felt 'insecure at home, so I need to get out and meet people. [The forum] makes me feel positive about myself'. Overall, parents who had participated seemed to value the forums and their work, and saw benefits both for themselves and for their children. As one parent said, 'I think that my contribution is welcomed and accepted and it is useful to find out what is going on.'

Programme boards

All six SSLPs had programme boards which met every four to six weeks with responsibility for strategic and operational issues. In theory, these boards should comprise six parent representatives, six statutory sector professionals and six representatives from the voluntary sector. In practice, some programmes had experienced difficulty recruiting sufficient numbers of parents. One programme had only two local parents serving at the time of our research, and this was said to have posed considerable problems for the transfer of information between the board and the parents' forum.

Recruitment to the board was generally through word of mouth, or nomination – either self-nomination or by a member of the parents' forum. Only one programme had held elections for membership. More usually, parents volunteered to step down or moved on naturally after serving for a year or two, making way for new parents to take their place.

Managers recognised that for many parents, the programme board could be 'heavy' and governance held little or no interest. In addition, the formality of the board could be overwhelming for parents with little experience of committees. Such parents risked feeling 'thrown in at the deep end' with jargon, paperwork and procedures. One parent summed up her experience:

> It's hard, they have a professional, and he's really nice, but it's just no one understands what he's talking about. He speaks great, I think he writes speeches for the MPs in the House of Commons, but I'm thinking, it's no good here, we're parents from London.

The need for parental support and training for participation was acknowledged by Sure Start workers, particularly as preparation for the programme boards. However, the cost in terms of time and resources could be high, with no assurance that active board membership would necessarily follow.

Only one-quarter of the parents interviewed knew what the programme board was. More than half had never heard of it, even more among those for whom English was not the first language. Nevertheless, just over one-quarter of parents interviewed said that they would be interested in joining.

Perceived value of parental involvement

Parents, staff and representatives of linked organisations were consistent in seeing benefits for parents and children from involvement at all levels in Sure Start programmes. The most commonly cited personal benefits for parents related to mood (47/60), making friends (46/60), parenting skills (41/60), confidence (41/60), relationships with children (40/60), coping with stress (38/60), access to services (30/60) and access to childcare (30/60). One father described the comfort of 'just knowing there's a place on the end of a phone, a centre you can drop into'.

Almost all parents identified ways in which involvement in Sure Start had helped their children. The most commonly described benefits for children were access to activities and new experiences (50/60), supporting knowledge and learning (45/60), developing confidence and social skills (43/60), and improving behaviour (34/60).

One mother who had suffered from severe postnatal depression described her son's progress at a SSLP respite crèche: 'He's a lot calmer and more intelligent, a different child from five months ago. He's learned from being with others and it gives me a break'. Involvement in Sure Start had got her out of the home, she said, and involved her in activities with other parents. Another parent looked back to her earlier, pre-Sure Start experience with her first child, maintaining that she would 'crack now without it'. After engaging in several activities for herself and her child, she had been encouraged by the employment and training worker to apply for a college place to study childcare, with the promise of help from Sure Start with her own childcare if necessary.

Staff considered that parents had gained skills and self-confidence from their involvement with the programme. Some parents had progressed along the continuum of involvement, moving from engagement in activities to attending the parents' forum, and subsequently serving on the programme board or engaging with other volunteering, training or employment opportunities.

All programmes had changed or developed their services in response to parents' wishes or suggestions. Parents had come with ideas and expertise, and were said by workers to have made a real contribution. A manager referred to the way that parent involvement demonstrates to other organisations the value of having users in developing and planning services; they have perhaps lots of expertise, and often they come up with much better ideas'. The potential exists to empower parents and build their capacity through giving them a sense of ownership of the programme, although as one manager pointed out, 'The balance needs to be right between supporting, empowering and doing it for them, and that is not easy'.

Developing parent involvement in Children's Centres

The six SSLPs that took part in this evaluation had evidently succeeded in engaging parents from a range of socioeconomic and ethnic backgrounds, and both parents and staff interviewed saw significant benefits from parent participation. Nonetheless, the findings indicated scope for improvement in terms of the programmes' ability to reach all sectors of the local community, as well as the potential to improve the processes by which parents were informed about and subsequently became engaged in activities at all levels.

The government's ongoing commitment to bottom-up inter-agency working (Department for Education and Skills 2003; HM Treasury 2004; Sure Start 2005a; Sure Start 2005b) raises questions about the development of parent involvement in the future Children's Centres. Can Sure Start's tradition of parent involvement be extended and maintained in future? As control of the new Children's Centres passes to the local authorities, fears have been expressed that Sure Start's tradition of bottom-up local working, building on community strengths and responding to local preferences, may become lost (Coote 2005; Glass 2005).

The research described here indicated that Sure Start workers and professionals such as health visitors have a key role to play in promoting parent involvement at all points on the continuum, but particularly in engaging hard-to-reach groups. In line with the National Evaluation of Sure Start (2005a, p.155; 2005b, p.15), our evaluation indicated that outreach was fundamental to engaging all members of the community, and particularly for users defined as 'facilitated' (needing more encouragement) or 'conditional' (parents who take up services if specific conditions are met) (National Evaluation of Sure Start 2005a, p.95; Tunstill et al. 2005b, p.164).

The incorporation of bottom-up values, mediated via parental involvement, must be consistent with any nationally imposed targets, posing a challenge for management (Bagley, Ackerley and Rattray 2004). To this end, the purpose and function of parent involvement must be clarified within partnerships. What is involvement is for? Who it is for? How can it be achieved? What criteria define its success? Such clarity will be critical for the expansion of parent involvement, implicit in the Children's Centre programme.

A further challenge relates to the balance of mainstreaming against the local determination of services. The experience of the SSLPs evaluated here indicates that consultation with parents needs to be extended, and awareness of groups like the parents' forum and dissemination of feedback must be developed. However, the forum should not be relied upon as a primary means of representing parents' views. Alternative models of consultation should be explored, such as using stay and play sessions to gather views and provide information about service development.

To ensure parental involvement in the governance of Children's Centres, Sure Start workers will again have a vital part to play in ensuring that the range of parents using services are represented, not just those whose professional or cultural backgrounds enable participation. Getting people actively involved in governance is difficult (Cook 2002; Gustafsson and Driver 2005). Recruitment, training and support for parents must be ongoing, particularly as the group is always moving on, to ensure a supply of parents willing – and adequately prepared – to participate. If the Children's Centre programme is committed to parental representation on boards, funding and strategic support for training and for dedicated parental involvement workers must be prioritised. A helpful parallel may be drawn with the work of school governors, which is managed locally (at a schools level), with support and training organised and delivered at a local authority level. (School governors are said to be the largest volunteer force in the UK, with approximately 1% of the adult population serving in this capacity at any one time (Governornet 2006)).

In the new Children's Centres, resources are likely to be at a level below that of Sure Start funding. For them to succeed in delivering effective and representative parental involvement, this work must have strategic priority and adequate dedicated resources.

Implications for Children's Centres

- Sure Start workers and other professionals have a key role to play in promoting parental involvement, particularly in engaging hard-to-reach groups; outreach is fundamental to engaging all members of the community.

- If the Children's Centre programme is committed to parental representation on boards, funding and strategic support for training and for dedicated parental involvement workers must be prioritised.

- Consultation with parents should be extended and alternative; less formal, models of consultation should be explored.

References

Arnstein, S.R. (1969) 'A ladder of citizen participation.' *Journal of the American Planning Association* 35, 4, 216–224.

Bagley, C., Ackerley, C. L. and Rattray, J. (2004) 'Social exclusion, Sure Start and organizational social capital: evaluating inter-disciplinary multi-agency working in an education and health work programme.' *Journal of Education Policy 19*, 5, 595–607.

Boddy, J., McQuail, S. and Wigfall, V. (2005) *Evaluation of Family Support and Parental Involvement in Local Programmes.* Unpublished report to Sure Start Islington.

Cook, D. (2002) 'Consultation for a change? Engaging users and communities in the policy process.' *Social Policy and Administration 36*, 5, 516–531.

Coote, A. (2005) 'But does Sure Start work?' *Society Guardian*, 19 January 2005.

Department for Education and Skills (2003) *Every Child Matters.* Cm 5860. London: The Stationery Office.

Eisenstadt, N. (2002) 'Sure Start: Key principles and ethos.' *Child: Care, Health and Development 28*, 1, 3–4.

Glass, N. (2005) 'Surely some mistake.' *Society Guardian*, 5 January 2005.

Governornet (2006) *Become a School Governor at This School.* www.governornet.co.uk/linkattachments/infosheets_1.doc, accessed on 10 October 2007.

Gustafsson, U. and Driver, D. (2005) 'Parents, power and public participation: Sure Start, an experiment in New Labour governance.' *Social Policy and Administration 39*, 5, 528–543.

Hart, R. (1992) *Children's Participation from Tokenism to Citizenship.* Florence: UNICEF.

HM Treasury (2004) *Choice for Parents, the Best Start for Children: A Ten-year Strategy for Childcare.* London: HM Treasury.

Kempson, E. and Whyley, C. (1999) *Kept Out or Opted Out? Understanding and Combating Financial Exclusion.* Bristol: The Policy Press.

National Evaluation of Sure Start (2005a) *Implementing Sure Start Local Programmes: An In-depth Study.* Research Report NESS/2005/FR/007. Nottingham: DfES.

National Evaluation of Sure Start (2005b) *Implementing Sure Start Local Programmes: An Integrated Overview of the First Four Years.* Research Report NESS/2005/FR/010. Nottingham: DfES.

Office of the Deputy Prime Minister (ODPM) (2004) *English Indices of Deprivation* (Revised). London: HMSO.

Office for National Statistics (2001) *Census 2001.* Available at www.statistics.gov.uk/census 2001/profiles/00AU-A.asp, accessed in October 2006.

Sanderson, I. (2002) 'Access to Services.' In Percy-Smith, J. (ed.) *Policy Responses to Social Exclusion: Towards Inclusion?* Maidenhead: Open University Press.

Sure Start (2005a) *Ten Year Strategy for Childcare: Guidance for Local Authorities.* London: Sure Start Unit. www.surestart.gov.uk/_doc/P0001651.pdf, accessed on 10 October 2006.

Sure Start (2005b) *A Sure Start Children's Centre for Every Community: Phase 2 Planning Guidance (2006–08). London: Sure Start Unit.* Available at www.surestart.gov.uk/_doc/ P0000457.doc, accessed on 10 October 2007.

Tunstill, J., Meadows, P., Allnock, D., Akhurst, S. and Garbers, C. (2005a) *Implementing Sure Start Local Programmes: An Integrated Overview of the First Four Years, National Evaluation Summary.* London: Sure Start Unit.

Tunstill, J., Allnock, D., Akhurst, S. and Garbers, C. (2005b) 'Sure Start Local Programmes: Implications of Case Study Data from the National Evaluation of Sure Start.' *Children and Society 19*, 158–171.

Chapter 10

Partnership between Parents and Professionals

Pamela Graham

Towards the latter part of the twentieth century there was a considerable shift towards partnership between parents and professionals, both within the legal and statutory framework and within different fields of practice. Today, the belief that early childhood programmes are more likely to succeed with effective parental involvement is taken for granted. However, what is meant by 'partnership with parents' can be contested and who is represented by the term 'professional' seems to be a matter of opinion. It could be argued that parenting itself is a profession.

Many models and typologies of partnership and participation fail to give weight to the dynamic aspect of the parent–professional relationship or to the subtle messages that can be and are transmitted from professionals to parents regarding their ability to parent (according to the accepted 'norm' of the given culture). These messages can, and do, leave parents feeling devalued in their role. This perceived power imbalance between parents and professionals is parallel to the power imbalance between children and adults. Just as children are conditioned to rely on parents or other adults during difficult periods, parents (quite possibly due to feelings of inadequacy) are conditioned to look to professionals for advice. This framework allows for comparison between the self-esteem of children as reflected to them by adults and the self-esteem of parents as reflected to them by professionals. The comparison between these relationships stems not from the belief that adults are 'childlike', nor does it intend to devalue professional expertise and knowledge. It stems from the belief that the power imbalance between children and adults and between parents and professionals is similar.

In many ways Sure Start was an innovative approach to the problems of inequity and limited opportunities for some groups of children and parents, yet in other ways it incorporated some taken-for-granted assumptions. One of these was that 'supporting' and 'involving' parents is unproblematic and revolves around technical processes such as communication, social activities and committee membership. There are many and more subtle aspects, however, to parental involvement and support. Not least of these is the centrality of parent–professional relationships as they are played out in relation to the children. The operation of Sure Start offered many opportunities to consider ways to address and improve partnership working and parent–professional relationships.

There is little doubt that parental interest and involvement in children's learning and development can enhance parent–child relationships and give children distinct advantages, but how that interest and involvement is valued and facilitated by those known as 'professionals' can also have a profound effect upon the self-esteem of all involved. There is nothing new here. In 1976 the Court Report (Court 1976) indicated a growing recognition that parents' confidence could be undermined by professional expertise. Pugh and De'Ath (1984) recommended that in education and support work with children, we should recognise and build upon parents' skills, abilities and experience. McConkey (1985) suggested that professionals should acknowledge the different roles of professionals and parents and Athey proposed that 'parents and professionals can help children separately or they can work together to the greater benefit of the children' (1990, p.66). The 1989 Children Act (Department of Health 1989) emphasised parental responsibility and referred to the parent–provider contract as an influencing factor in the quality of care for young children. The Parenting Forum, formed at the beginning of 1995, aimed 'to raise the awareness of the importance of parenting and its widespread impact on the personal, emotional, mental and educational development of children' (National Children's Bureau 1995).

When Labour came into power in May 1997, they pledged to invest heavily in early years care and education. Beginning with the National Childcare Strategy (Department for Education and Skills 2001), several major initiatives were introduced, many of which formed the basis for the inordinate amount of current initiatives which purport to work in partnership with parents. The Curriculum Guidance for the Foundation Stage stated that 'Parents and practitioners should work together in an atmosphere of mutual respect within which children can have security and confidence' (Department for Education and Employment 2000, p.11). The Sure Start initiative declared a commitment to supporting parents. The Children's Centre programme builds upon the work of Sure Start and is based on the concept that the provision of integrated services is key to determining positive outcomes for children and parents. The 2004 Children Act provides the legal framework for the current programme of reform set out in the green paper *Every Child Matters* (Department for Education and Skills 2003). This confirmed that some parents do not receive the necessary support to fulfil their parenting role, and clearly acknowledges the undeniable link between effective parenting and the well-being of children and young people: 'As the one constant in a child or young person's life, parents are absolutely key to promoting positive outcomes and ensuring that children and young people achieve their potential'.

Influences on parental self-esteem

Low self-esteem is a characteristic recognised in many parents. It may be impossible to know how much of it is individualistic, how much of it is a result of social policies which create dependency, how much has been reinforced by a paternalistic culture in which women are expected to nurture and protect their children, or how much it relates to unrealistic expectations of children. There are so many possible contributing factors. Parental self-esteem clearly influences parenting behaviours. Levels of parental self-esteem have been linked to the quality of parent–child interactions and low self-esteem linked to the maltreatment of children. Campion suggested that in order to provide effective childcare we need to tackle low maternal self-esteem. She identified recurring themes in literature on parents labelled as 'inadequate' or 'unfit': 'emotional immaturity, social isolation, low self-image and unreal expectations of children' and reflected upon how these labels can 'add to their social isolation and low self-esteem with further implications for their capacity to care for their children' (Campion 1995, p.33).

It seems reasonable to suggest that comparisons can be drawn between the self-esteem of children as reflected to them by their parents and the self-esteem of parents as reflected to them by professionals. Kitzinger and Kitzinger suggested that in order for children's self-esteem to develop, 'adults have to surrender some of their power and have to allow children to choose between alternatives, to experience some self-direction in their daily lives and not to be under the control of adults' (Kitzinger and Kitzinger 1990, p.95). In order for parents' self-esteem to develop and parent–child relationships to develop it may be that professionals have to afford parents similar autonomy.

Professional beliefs and values

Working in genuine partnership is dependent upon shared beliefs and values, or at least upon mutual understanding and respect between partners who differ. A number of 'clashes' between organisations, between different professionals and between parents and professionals were evident in the data, with subtle messages about 'good parenting' and 'good behaviour', many with unrealistic expectations of children, being transmitted from a wide range of sources. With the increasing popularity of 'parenting programmes' it is time to consider seriously the impact that these messages have on the self-esteem of participating parents and ultimately on the self-esteem of children.

The sheer number of training packs on 'parenting skills' and 'child management' is overwhelming. Many claim to improve parent–child relationships but are actually advertised as packs for professionals who work with parents.

Such terminology reinforces the 'professionals know best' culture and supports the argument that some types of professional intervention can do more harm than good.

When concerns are raised regarding parenting skills, many questions need to be answered about why we believe certain parents would benefit from parenting programmes, how they feel about participating and how they feel about professionals wanting them to change. The well motivated parent, who identifies areas of parenting they would like to explore, clearly needs something completely different from the parent emerging from the child protection process who may feel pressurised to show professionals that they want to be a 'good' parent, or a socially isolated parent craving contact with understanding adults. And there are so many 'what ifs'. What if parents who have attended parenting courses which claim to turn them into 'competent' or 'better parents' – maybe even providing them with certificates to prove it – have a domestic crisis or a run of challenging interactions with their children? Will they cope because their certificate says they can? Or will a sense of failure overwhelm them? What if a facilitator's idea of the child's best interests is at odds with a parent's? Interestingly, parents who also carry the 'professional' label have identified feeling vulnerable in the presence of colleagues when parenting is under the spotlight.

In order to encourage parents to be involved in their children's development and learning there needs to be genuine mutual respect and trust. However, this depends very much upon the beliefs, values, skills and priorities of both professionals and parents. Children and adults alike need to be emotionally nurtured. We know that children of emotionally healthy adults are likely to be emotionally healthy as children and as parents of the future. Professionals have a huge responsibility to acknowledge this in their work.

The status of children and its impact on parenting

The different rights and responsibilities attributed to adults and children in the UK suggest that the status of childhood is considered (by some) to be a separate and somehow inferior stage to adulthood. Clues about the status and importance of children are reflected in the nature and number of services available and in the expectations on those who work within them. Each service works to slightly different priorities and rules and holds different beliefs about partnership with parents. Some services aim to free more women to go out to work, others aim to 'socialise' children or 'prepare them for school'. Some services are welfare services clearly targeted to meet the needs of children and parents with 'social problems'. It is important to question whose beliefs and ideas about children and parents are reflected in these services and how they influence partnership with parents.

Different paradigms of care and control for children and families influence different systems and professions in different ways. Within each paradigm there will be a desirable outcome which may contradict the core values of the family or indeed those of other systems and professions. Many children and families are influenced by more than one paradigm, which can only serve to confuse. Stainton-Rogers bases two images of children – 'the innocent and wholesome child' and 'the wicked and sinful child' – on two discourses: the 'discourse of welfare' and the 'discourse of control'. She suggests that the first discourse informs UK social policy and legislation for young children and is based upon the assumptions that children 'are entitled to a good childhood and that they need protection'. The second discourse 'informs education policy towards children' and is based upon 'the assumption that children lack self-control and need to be regulated' (Stainton-Rogers *et al.* 2001, p.30). These discourses can be identified clearly in our early childhood services.

Many parents (and non-parent adults) truly believe that children should neither question nor challenge them. One result of this is children becoming conditioned to 'do as they are told' and to conform to adults' expectations whilst suppressing their natural creativity, curiosity and spontaneity. This can result in a range of misunderstandings between parents and children, parents and professionals, and children and professionals in many combinations. Add these misunderstandings to other common stresses, such as unstable adult relationships, poor housing, low income or unemployment, and it could be suggested that the chances of deterioration in the parent–child relationship seem set to increase unless parents are truly empowered to change things.

Professionals, even with the very best intentions, can cause parents to be filled with doubt about their ability to 'do the right thing'. Anna, mother of Ali (three years), described her experiences during Ali's first three months at nursery when he regularly wet his pants:

> I felt awful, it was mainly the way the staff were not exactly interrogating, but asking me all the time about it. They asked if everything was OK at home. They asked questions about how I was toilet training him. It made me think I'd done something wrong. Then when he stopped they said not to worry because it was quite common, and I thought "Well why couldn't you have told me that before?" I was so upset and so was he. I felt like a really bad mother.

Julie (mother of three children aged between two and seven years) talked about early years practitioners (who when interviewed viewed their approach as 'empowering'): 'Sometimes they make me feel like I'm doing it right and sometimes they make me feel like I'm doing something wrong. It's nice when they ask my opinions'.

Margy (mother of four children aged between 11 months and nine years) described her experiences following regular parent workshops during which the emphasis was on building on the strengths of both parents and children: 'I think I listen to them [children] more and show an interest in what they do now. I try to look at things from their point of view instead of just assuming they understand' (Graham 2002, p.23).

The involvement of parents in Sure Start programmes

By its very nature, much of Sure Start's work has been to do with parenting. The changing roles of mothers and fathers, particularly in relation to employment opportunities, have presented challenges to many of the long established beliefs and attitudes of parents and practitioners, and have required a drastic overhaul of early years services. Sure Start's attention to the importance of the parenting role, particularly its impact upon the social, emotional and educational development of the child, offered numerous opportunities for contact with parents who had previously failed to engage with mainstream services. In all of the programmes evaluated, it was apparent that various health and social care professionals were able to build relationships with these families, and to establish the type of contact that other mainstream professionals had tried in vain to establish. This often relied upon contact in different types of contexts, engaging in different types of initiatives. However, a small but significant number of professionals seemed uncomfortable with the expectation that they should participate in social events with children and parents. They believed that it somehow diminished their professional authority.

Recent government initiatives with seemingly contradictory messages have, at times, confused both professionals and parents. For example, Sure Start's remit to work with parents and children to establish good parent–child relationships and the government's 'welfare to work' initiative left some wondering whether 'good' parents should go out to work to provide for their children or stay at home and spend quality time with their children. Furthermore, time-limited targets restricted opportunities to develop the relationships necessary to achieve ultimate goals.

Some concern was expressed about the level and nature of parental engagement and of Sure Start's expectations of parents. Whilst professionals agreed that the concept of parental involvement is good, their concerns were about the amount of training that is needed to bring parents to a level where they are able to make properly formulated decisions, and the possible danger of parents becoming disenchanted if they did not feel sufficiently listened to.

'Moving parents on' was also raised as a sensitive issue. Parents identified the need for something satisfying to move on to once their children were beyond the age of the services. This is a common problem for organisations that rely upon voluntary contribution for organisational and management purposes. If a group of parents become identified within the community as having a certain role in a project, it becomes difficult to involve new parents without pushing the originals out. Parent interviewees who were involved in a more active capacity felt that in order for new parents to be confident enough to become parent representatives in meetings or as members of management groups, they should be trained or 'apprenticed' to current parent representatives. As one parent pointed out:

> New parents would be scared. It was hard in the beginning – for parents and professionals. We were always scared to speak up in meetings. You can get walked all over. Now we need parents with confidence. They have to speak up for others. There should be parent training available for management, like we've had equal opportunities training for interviewing.

In some programmes there was an expectation that parents should attend meetings and many did so willingly. One parent, however, raised the issue of inequity and questioned whether professionals could be exploiting parents to further their own careers.

Professional identity, teamwork and 'innovative practice'

In response to recent government policy there have been a significant number of changes all of which have required, and will require further, changes to practice for those professionals who work with parents in integrated children's services. 'Innovative practice' has been mentioned time and again both locally and nationally in relation to Sure Start. In relation to innovative activities and meeting government targets, the ability to pilot, take risks, experiment and cope with 'failures' as well as 'successes' appears to emerge as one of the key requirements of a successful Sure Start practitioner. This way of working requires high levels of confidence, especially for those practitioners who have come from more 'traditional' roles.

Successful innovative practice appears to be about how effective a team is at interpreting current community need and investing time and resources to setting up and delivering packages which are culturally appropriate and which involve and empower parents and community representatives. Whilst there was clear evidence of a deep commitment to wanting to work as a team, there were also instances of practitioners feeling very cautious about relinquishing 'professional autonomy'. There seems to be an indication from some professionals that maintaining a specialism whilst working in a multidisciplinary way is important. Getting some parents and children involved with Sure Start does initially seem to rely upon 'traditional' contacts with defined professionals such as health visitors, family support workers and speech and language therapists. One evaluation identified that staff did not feel particularly 'fixed' in their roles and that Sure Start by its very nature had provided opportunities for a move towards innovative roles. It was suggested that some staff were more 'inclined towards working with parents' than others, depending on their previous professional experience, the culture of their own agency and even their personality. It was acknowledged that 'new and innovative ways' of working might have implications for the maintenance of the professional's registration with the relevant professional body.

Cost-effectiveness

In some programmes, there were concerns about the relatively small numbers of parents involved in some of the programme's activities. This was clearly a 'cost-effectiveness' issue. When trying to establish the best way to use time and resources in order to meet targets, the tensions between providing innovative services which are tailored to community needs and being 'cost-effective' will always be there, at least as long as success is measured in monetary terms.

Schon (1991) explored professional practice and noted that the 'real' problems requiring solutions do not have simple research-based answers. In the topography of practice they do not occupy the 'firm, hard ground' but demand that practitioners struggle in the 'swampy lowlands', finding and testing out their own solutions. This takes time and resources. Initial enthusiasm and understandable naivety means that in partnership work with parents, errors may have to be made and new avenues may have to be explored.

The way forward

Evidence from the data suggested that staffing and organisational structures alongside complex management and supervision issues often hindered integrated working and the establishment of effective communication channels between management, practitioners and ultimately parents. Yet Sure Start continued to evolve and to be a catalyst for what appears to have been relentless change. This has been achieved through the determination and flexibility of parents and professionals on the ground, who held on to the Sure Start vision.

True progression will not only rely upon the development of a shared vision with shared policies and strategies at an organisational level, but it will also require the development of shared understandings between everyone involved in services for children and families. There is a clear way forward set out in *Every Child Matters* (Department for Education and Skills 2003) and *The National Service Framework* (Department of Health 2004) and with the move into the Children's Centre era there will be many opportunities to challenge deficit models of parenting, raise aspirations and rebalance the power relationships between professions and between parents and professionals.

Implications for Children's Centres

- We need to ensure that the beliefs and values underpinning practice in every Children's Centre are transparent and do not promote the 'professionals know best' culture that has thus hindered partnership working in the past.

- As we work towards integration, we need to find ways of valuing the expertise of all parents and practitioners (from every professional heritage), yet at the same time develop shared understandings of how to work together to meet the needs of children and families.

- Services for children and families have been subject to unprecedented change over the last decade; it is time to slow down and allow these new ways of working to embed, develop and produce the desired results.

Summary

This chapter has explored some of the nuances in parent–professional partnerships and their potential impact on the lives of parents and young children. The data were collected between 2001 and 2006 and illustrate some of the complex issues involved in this debate. They were taken from the author's own research and nine Sure Start Local Programme evaluations carried out in the North of England, which for contractual and ethical reasons have not been identified. The methodologies employed were a combination of fieldwork and desk-based techniques. Approximately 50 days were spent in each site consulting and collecting data. The data itself comprised questionnaires (co-constructed and administered by local people), interviews, focus groups, case studies and documentary data, including minutes of meetings, local statistics and monthly reach information. Observation of all sites was conducted at regular intervals throughout each year. The data were triangulated and the qualitative elements were coded according to observed processes and concept development (Glaser and Strauss 1967).

References

Athey, C. (1990) *Extending Thought in Young Children.* London: Paul Chapman.

Campion, M.J. (1995) *Who's Fit to Be a Parent?* London: Routledge.

Court, S.D.M. (1976) *Fit for the Future. The Report of the Committee on Child Health Services.* London: HMSO.

Department for Education and Employment (2000) *Curriculum Guidance for the Foundation Stage.* London: Qualifications and Curriculum Authority.

Department for Education and Skills (2001) *The National Childcare Strategy.* London: DfES.

Department for Education and Skills (2003) *Every Child Matters.* London: DfES.
    www.everychildmatters.gov.uk/participation/faq/, accessed on 9 November 2007.

Department of Health (1989) *The Children Act 1989.* London: HMSO.

Department of Health (2004) *National Service Framework for Children, Young People and Maternity Services.* London: DoH.

Glaser, B. and Strauss, A. (1967) *The Discovery of Grounded Theory.* Chicago, IL: Aldine.

Graham, P. (2002) Section in J. Santer (ed.) *Young Children Learning 1.* Newcastle: Newcastle University.

Kitzinger, S. and Kitzinger, C. (1990) *Talking with Children about Things that Matter.* London: Pandora.

National Children's Bureau (1995) *The Parenting Forum Newsletter, 1.* London: National Childhood Bureau.

McConkey, R. (1985) *Working with Parents – A Practical Guide for Teachers and Therapists.* Kent: Croom Helm Ltd.

Pugh, G. and De'Ath, E. (1984) *The Needs of Parents.* Basingstoke: MacMillan.

Schon, D. (1991) *The Reflective Practitioner: How Professionals Think in Action.* Aldershot: Avebury.

Stainton-Rogers, W. (2001) 'Constructing childhood, constructing child concern.' In P. Foley, J. Roche and S. Tucker *Children in Society: Contemporary Theory, Policy and Practice.* Basingstoke: Palgrave in association with The Open University.

Chapter 11

Local Programmes and Social Services: Lessons in Partnership

Michaela Griffin and John Carpenter

Sure Start Local Programmes (SSLPs) have been held up by the Department for Education and Skills (now the Department for Children, Schools and Families) as a model for the development of children's services in England. In particular, the value and importance of partnership working has been emphasised. The study described in this chapter examined the relationships between eight SSLPs and four local authorities with social services responsibilities (Social Services Departments (SSDs)). It investigated how they worked together to provide preventative services to children under four years and examined the impacts. Enablers and barriers to partnerships are discussed in terms of organisational, cultural and professional, and contextual issues.

Background

The Children Act 2004 re-emphasised the importance of partnership in children's services. The policy changes recognised that the needs of children and families do not fit within organisational boundaries and imposed a duty on key agencies to work together. Hudson (2005) characterised the mode of governance presented as 'whole systems working', while identifying omissions and contradictions within the government's approach that would create problems for those charged with the implementation of the Act. In terms of the reshaping of children's services, SSLPs were held up as a model for partnership.

The literature provides frameworks for the analysis of the process of joint working and progression in the development of partnerships. For example, Frost (2005, p.13) proposed a four-level hierarchical model, progressing from 'cooperation', through to 'collaboration' – where services plan together to meet common outcomes, to systematic 'coordination' of services to meet shared and agreed goals, and finally to 'merger/integration' to become one organisation. In a complementary fashion, Cameron and Lart's (2003) systematic review offered a comparative framework for identifying what helps and what hinders joint working in terms of organisational, cultural and professional, and contextual issues.

The National Evaluation of Sure Start (NESS) 'Implementation Module' (Tunstill *et al.* 2005) involved an exploration of SSLPs and the management of partnerships. These researchers concluded that SSLPs 'face a complex task in building programme partnerships...' (p.161). They identified three key issues:

1. The extent to which leadership and management were effective in helping staff transcend traditional boundaries.

2. The value of clearly defined protocols governing the relationship between the partnership and the lead/accountable body.

3. The importance of engaging professionals with different perspectives and experiences in strategy development.

This chapter develops the findings from the NESS study through a set of case studies of SSLPs and their relationships with one of their key partners: local authorities with social services responsibilities (SSDs). The analysis was conducted in the light of the frameworks offered by Frost (2005) and Cameron and Lart (2003).

Aims

The aim of this study, then, was to examine the relationships between SSLPs and SSDs. In this way, we hoped to identify some lessons for the further development of partnerships in children's services.

Method

The study took place in four SSD areas in the northeast of England in 2004 and focused on two established and fully operational SSLPs in each area. Thirty-six front-line practitioners and managers from Sure Start and social services were invited to theorise about, and comment on, their experiences and expectations of the development of integrated services for children and to identify any benefits they perceived from partnerships. The interviews were analysed thematically.

Findings

Sure Start programmes tried to 'reach out' to whole neighbourhoods. In each of the areas studied, they aimed to offer non-stigmatising, universal services, from family-friendly local centres. They sought to develop long-term relationships with families and communities to identify and respond to risks early.

> We are well established and well trusted within the community. So we get neighbours coming to us with concerns who would not go to social services... (SSLP manager, Area 1)

All of the programmes also worked with families to remove children from social work caseloads or the child protection register. However, the extent to which this was done in partnership with social services varied across the areas.

Several participants argued that Sure Start was addressing gaps in provision that had opened up with the refocusing of social work practice on short-term intervention and the most 'vulnerable' children and families (translated as families where there was concern about child neglect and abuse) instead of prevention through relationships with people and communities. They considered that Sure Start was needed because the nature of social services work had changed with the need to prioritise and ration resources. The issue identified was not lack of coordination between agencies, but lack of funding.

Experiences of joint working

Local politics and the history of policy developments, together with social factors in each of the areas, influenced the expectations and responses of those involved in the development of joint working arrangements in services for families and children. Social services' involvement with Sure Start at the partnership board level varied across the case study programmes, but this did not predict the effectiveness of joint working at the levels of operational management, service development and delivery.

In Area 1 there was an established shared protocol between Sure Start and social services for responding to the needs of children and families. Social services funded Sure Start posts and resources were shared, including day care. Practitioners and managers trained together. Sure Start health visitors contributed to social services' core assessments.

In Area 4, there was an agreed referral and allocation process, and managers from social services and local programmes met regularly. Day care and training resources were pooled. However, there were few opportunities for collaboration in service development and delivery.

Joint working arrangements were at an early stage of development in Area 2, with social services managers only recently having joined Partnership Boards. There were no agreed referral procedures and no pooling of resources.

Experiences differed between the programmes in Area 3. Programme 3a had always enjoyed regular involvement from social services managers, and social services funded Sure Start posts. Practitioners jointly ran some groups and organised events. However, there were no agreed referral procedures. Programme 3b had less involvement from social services than Programme 3a had, when it was becoming established. However, the relationship had improved during the previous year. There were still no social services funded posts in programme 3b, but the SSD and the SSLP were piloting a common assessment and database, with staff training together.

Joint working with individual families was developing in some areas. In Areas 1 and 4, examples were cited of successful collaboration in casework, including joint assessments and coordinated packages of support. In Areas 2 and 3, SSD and SSLP practitioners only liaised informally about individual families. Social workers sometimes contacted SSLPs to inquire about services for families whose needs did not meet social services' eligibility criteria, but did not routinely refer families.

Variations in the extent of joint working across the eight programmes are summarised in Table 11.1 based on the hierarchical model proposed by Frost (2005). Only Areas 1 and 4 had reached the third level of 'coordination', where services worked together in a planned and systematic way towards shared goals. In Area 2, the 'partners' were just moving from working in parallel, with only ad hoc reference to each other about individual 'cases', to Frost's first level of 'cooperation', where complementary services are provided by agencies, working separately towards consistent goals. In Area 3, joint working had developed at different paces. Collaboration, where services plan together, addressing duplication and gaps in services towards common outcomes, was more established between one SSLP (3a) and social services, than the other (3b). These differences, within one authority, were attributed to local historical and social factors, in particular, the relationships between people in partner agencies and past experience and expectations of multi-agency initiatives.

The development of joint working proved, however, to be more complex than Frost's model allowed, with variation in progress within programmes, between strategic developments and operational management, service delivery and individual casework. In response to the Children Act 2004, all areas were moving up to Frost's (2005) fourth level strategically, through integration of education and social services, into one local authority department. Area 2 had already merged all council services for children and young people into a 'Lifelong Learning' directorate, the lead partner for Sure Start, yet there was no joint working in service delivery. This demonstrated the 'top-down' implementation problem identified by Hudson (2005); a merger at the strategic level does not guarantee integration at the front-line.

What helped and what hindered joint working?
Cameron and Lart (2003) identified three broad groups of issues that influenced the effectiveness of joint working arrangements. They were organisational, cultural and professional, and contextual. Participants' accounts will be considered under these headings, with other analytical tools acknowledged where relevant.

Table 11.1 Joint working in the four areas: Using Frost's (2005) 'levels of development'

Area	Cooperation	Collaboration	Coordination	Integration
Area 1			Operational Management and Strategic Management	Individual Casework and Service Delivery
Area 2	Individual Casework and Service Delivery	Operational Management		Strategic Management
Area 3a		Individual Casework and Service Delivery	Operational Management and Strategic Management	
Area 3b	Individual Casework	Service Delivery and Operational Management	Strategic Management	
Area 4	Service Delivery	Individual Casework	Operational Management and Strategic Management	

ORGANISATIONAL ISSUES

Participants from both social services and Sure Start said that they shared a common objective of promoting the welfare of children. Nevertheless, they agreed that their priorities were different. For social services, the priority was protecting the most 'vulnerable' children and therefore working with the minority of families in greatest need or at greatest risk. For Sure Start, the priority was all families in historically disadvantaged areas. This divergence was also identified in the national study (Tunstill *et al.* 2005). Where joint working seemed strongest, in Areas 1 and 4, participants described a shared vision. All participants had positive expectations about the development of shared assessments and information systems, and coordinated responses tiered to the level of concern, as proposed in *Every Child Matters* (HM Treasury 2003). However, several feared that, with the move to integrated children's services, educational objectives might take priority over those of health and social services, undermining the progress already achieved in joint working. Some participants thought that the imposition of certain government objectives, particularly encouraging parents into employment, could alienate the families that all partners most wanted to help. Theoretical critics of New Labour's social policy and its assumption that 'joined-up' working is a 'good thing' of itself (Allen 2003; Frost 2005; Kidger 2004; Rummery 2002) would recognise these concerns about the power imbalance between agencies and the apparent removal of choice from parents.

There was an association between the Partnership Board arrangements and the strength of joint working at the operational level in Area 4, where social services was the lead partner. However, in other areas the association was mediated through local politics, past experiences and expectations of policy change, and established relationships. In Area 1, where joint working was also strong, different partners (the Primary Care Trust and the local authority) led the programmes. In Area 3, Programme A had originally been led by social services and the manager had enjoyed the active support of social services management. Programme 3b had originally been led by a voluntary organisation and social services had only recently become involved. Although the lead partner for the Area 2 programmes was the council's merged 'Lifelong Learning' department, front-line joint working with social services was in its infancy. Strategic support and commitment from senior managers were identified as underpinning joint working arrangements in Areas 1 and 4 and in Programme 3a. Success was frequently attributed to the influence of key managers and their ability to establish and sustain relationships with their counterparts in other agencies.

> Both the social services manager and the commissioning manager were likeminded and determined to go the extra mile. (Social work team manager)

Cameron and Lart (2003) stressed the importance of clearly identified roles and responsibilities, and joint working was most effective in Areas 1 and 4 where they were agreed. Managers in both areas regularly reviewed shared policies and procedures. Common understanding and agreement, on distinct and shared roles and responsibilities, were still to be achieved in Areas 2 and 3.

Legal, ethical and practical obstacles to sharing information were perceived to be major barriers in all areas. Yet information sharing emerged, from both Frost's (2005) and Cameron and Lart's (2003) reviews, as key to effective joint working. Regular, face-to-face and informal contact was associated with effective communication in both the reviews. Formal and informal communication varied across the programmes studied, and the ease and regularity of both differed with the strength of joint working. The more contact participants had with each other, the more inclined they were to seek and support further communication. Where contact was facilitated by co-location in shared accommodation, participants readily cited the advantages of being based together. Consequently there was general support for the idea of Children's Centres as buildings to accommodate practitioners from different agencies with responsibilities for children. However, the co-location of social workers within Sure Start Centres was controversial, with concerns expressed that their presence might 'stigmatise' the programmes.

Lack of capacity in social services was consistently identified as a major obstacle to effective joint working in all areas.

> The general feeling is that what obstructs joint work is lack of capacity in social services' teams to spare for anything extra. (SSLP manager)

Funding pressures and recruitment and retention problems were exacerbated by the conflicting demands on managers to participate in a range of 'initiatives' while managing excess demand for services. In Areas 2 and 3, social services managers thus explained why they had previously been unable to commit their time to Sure Start. Turnover and recruitment difficulties in SSLPs also presented problems in sustaining joint initiatives; these were exacerbated by short-term contracts and uncertainty about future funding.

Expectations of joint working, based on experience locally, affected the willingness of social services managers to get involved in partnerships. This was particularly the case in Area 3, where past experiences had initially given operational managers low expectations of Sure Start. Before the recent policy focus on partnerships, more voluntary sector partnerships and initiatives had been funded there than in the other authorities. However, their role had usually been transitory and perceived as disregarding the priorities of social services.

> Over the years social services felt powerless to influence the voluntary sector... A lot of the more experienced staff have seen projects like Sure Start come and go, over thirty years. (Social work team manager)

In contrast in Area 1, progress already achieved in joint working with the Primary Care Trust had contributed to participants' positive expectations of Sure Start.

The power imbalance between organisations and professionals was identified as an obstacle to joint working. Social services were perceived as the agency with statutory powers and responsibilities to force compliance from uncooperative parents. The status of social workers, compared with other professionals working with children, obstructed equal partnership in service delivery.

CULTURAL AND PROFESSIONAL ISSUES

The negative impact of professional and organisational stereotypes was evident from participants' accounts of discussions about the community's hostility to social workers and social services. The fear of stigmatising universal services by association with social workers meant they had been excluded from Sure Start delivery plans.

> Families generally regard their facilities positively because they are open to everybody and they are seen as supportive and non-threatening and *not* social services. We are known for taking children away, not for supporting families. (Social work team manager)

All the SSLPs had 'family support' staff, sometimes seconded by social services. However, none had qualified practitioners employed in social work roles and this was now generally recognised as a gap. In Area 1, the SSLPs wanted social workers to bring their skills to their teams, because parents unhappy about families being referred to social services would accept the involvement of social workers employed in the programmes. However, in Area 2, social services managers predicted that as children's services become integrated, local authority social workers would have to focus on statutory work, reinforcing current stereotypes and cultural and organisational barriers to joint working.

The universal nature of Sure Start services was an obstacle to effective collaboration for social services managers obliged to concentrate resources on those at greatest risk (c.f. Tunstill *et al.* 2005). That Sure Start works only with the consent and cooperation of families was regarded as another barrier to sharing priorities and values. Social services professionals were accustomed to grappling with the dilemma of reconciling the values of parental empowerment with the priority of protecting children. Although in principle agencies shared responsibilities for protecting children, social services managers believed that other agencies were reluctant to accept them in practice.

Cameron and Lart (2003) identified trust and respect as key ingredients in successful joint working and this was supported by Tunstill and colleagues (2005, p.161). Established relationships between staff in partner agencies helped.

> I was already local and understood their work, so I can talk to social services staff informally. (SSLP worker)

In Area 3, the historical distrust of partnerships (discussed above) did not obstruct joint working in Programme A, partly because the programme manager was already known and trusted by social services colleagues. Key post holders in Area 4 SSLPs were similarly respected locally. Pre-existing relationships between Sure Start staff and social services underpinned collaboration in Area 1.

Participants in all areas identified the potential benefits of shared training in promoting communication and understanding of respective roles and responsibilities – factors identified as significant to the development of effective partnerships (Cameron and Lart 2003; Frost 2005).

CONTEXTUAL ISSUES

Re-organisation of partner agencies that led to key personnel changes interrupted the development of relationships and mutual understanding in our study. Organisational instability was identified as undermining joint working by Cameron and Lart (2003) and so was financial uncertainty. Sure Start programmes appeared to be well-resourced initially to develop and promote new services. This provoked some resentment from staff in social services, where resources were increasingly rationed to meet needs and policy requirements. Yet the long-term funding of SSLPs seemed insecure, despite the Green Paper proposals (HM Treasury 2003).

Lack of coterminosity between social services' and SSLPs' areas of responsibility meant that where social service managers considered that most of their work came from outside the programme areas or age limits, joint working with SSLPs was not prioritised.

The impact of the government's 'modernisation' programme on social services managers' capacity was repeatedly highlighted as a major barrier to involvement in partnerships.

> But more and more initiatives impact on managers' capacity and time to spend working with partners. We have to revert to concentrating on core business. (Social work team manager)

Managers selected the initiatives to support, based on their own priorities. Uncertainty obstructed joint planning. Participants feared that policies would change before being fully implemented. Social services managers were not persuaded that partner agencies would be willing and able to share the responsibilities for statutory work. They foresaw the tensions and omissions, identified by Hudson (2005) in the 'whole systems approach', in the government's failure to oblige some key partners (GPs and schools) to cooperate. Even where joint working was strongest, there was concern that the government's policy objectives did not match local needs, resources and priorities. Like Dowling, Powell and Glendinning (2004), participants were unconvinced that the proposals for reform were pragmatic and evidence-based.

> Partnership and collaboration have not been the problem here. It's lack of clarity from government and the imposition of priorities that might not be those of the community. (Social work team manager)

Conclusions

Participants' accounts of the development of joint working indicated that it was influenced by their expectations and experiences of inter-agency partnerships locally, as well as central government policy. The factors that helped or hindered joint working, identified in Cameron and Lart's (2003) review, were relevant to each of the 'partnerships' studied. However, development did not follow a linear progression, as suggested by Frost's (2005) hierarchical model. Instead the complexity and contradictions in the 'whole systems' approach to children's services, predicted by Hudson (2005), were apparent as partnerships were stronger at some layers of the whole system than others.

Implications for Children's Centres

- Local experiences and expectations of partnerships between agencies should be taken into account in the planning and development of Children's Centres.

- Integration of services at the strategic management level does not guarantee effective joint working at the level of service delivery; clear protocols and agreements between agencies on referral processes, eligibility criteria and respective roles and responsibilities promote effective partnerships.

- The development of relationships facilitated by face-to-face contact, through joint training, meetings or shared accommodation, is important in the development of the trust, communication and mutual understanding required for successful collaboration in service planning, development and delivery.

Acknowledgements

The study was commissioned by the Department for Education and Skills (now the Department for Children, Schools and Families) and was conducted at the Durham Centre for Applied Social Research, Durham University. The conclusions do not necessarily represent the views of the then DfES. We would like to thank Jayne Moules, Director of the Regional Sure Start Unit, NorthEast and members of the project advisory group representing participating SSDs and Sure Start Local Programmes.

References

Allen, C. (2003) 'Desperately seeking fusion: on "joined up" thinking, "holistic practice" and the new economy of welfare professional power.' *British Journal of Sociology 54*, 287–306.

Cameron, A. and Lart, R. (2003) 'Factors promoting and obstacles hindering joint working: a systematic review of the research evidence.' *Journal of Integrated Care 11*, 9–17.

Dowling, B., Powell, M. and Glendinning, C. (2004) 'Conceptualising successful partnerships.' *Health and Social Care in the Community 12*, 309–317.

Frost, N. (2005) *Professionalism, Partnership and Joined-up Thinking*. Dartington: Research in Practice.

HM Treasury (2003) *Every Child Matters*, Cm5860. London: The Stationery Office.

Hudson, B. (2005) 'Partnership working and the children's services agenda: is it feasible?' *Journal of Integrated Care 13*, 7–12.

Kidger, J. (2004) 'Including young mothers: limitations to New Labour's strategy for supporting teenage parents.' *Critical Social Policy 24*, 291–311.

Rummery, K. (2002) 'Towards a theory of welfare partnerships.' In C. Glendinning, M. Powell and K. Rummery (eds) *Partnerships, New Labour and the Governance of Welfare*. Bristol: Policy Press.

Tunstill, J., Allnock, D., Akhurst, S., Garbers, C. and NESS Research Team (2005) 'Sure Start Local Programmes: implications of case study data from the National Evaluation of Sure Start.' *Children and Society 19*, 158–171.

Chapter 12

Perceptions of Statutory Service Providers of Local Programmes

Alison Edgley

Sure Start has been a central feature of government policy designed to promote partnerships and inter-agency working (McLaughlin 2004) in children's services. A more collaborative and integrated model of service delivery has underpinned a range of more recent policy initiatives from the Children Bill (House of Lords 2004), to *Every Child Matters* (Department for Education and Skills 2003), as well as *The National Service Framework for Children, Young People and Maternity Services* (Department of Health and Department for Education and Skills 2004), all of which aim to improve public services so they better meet the needs of children and young people. Sure Start then has been one element in a broader context of policy developments designed to address perceived gaps in service provision for children, by cultivating collaborative and integrated service provision.

By 2010, however, it is intended that Sure Start services will have become 'mainstreamed'. In 2004 the Treasury announced that every family should have easy access to integrated services through Children's Centres in their local community (HM Treasury 2004). This means that the 534 national Sure Start programmes will be extended to become part of local authority-run children's trusts through 3500 Children's Centres in every community (Department for Children, Schools and Families 2007). It is also intended that both the services and the ways of working characteristic of Sure Start are intended to permeate statutory service provision.

Sure Start, then, has had three features that distinguish it from mainstream statutory services. First, it has been targeted specifically at deprived families. Second, it is an agency designed to offer a range of services from a multi-professional team tailored to the particular needs of a community. Third, it is designed to be responsive to community needs, by involving parents in decisions about service provision through the Partnership Boards. Mainstreaming is intended to ensure that the Sure Start ethos is incorporated into statutory service provision. The government's agenda then is to ensure that mainstream statutory services adapt in ways that ensure they are integrated and responsive to need.

Aim

This study explored the perceptions of statutory service providers working in mainstream health, education and social welfare services about the impact of working with Sure Start.

Method

Semistructured interviews were conducted with 18 local professionals from mainstream statutory services between January and March 2005. The 18 statutory providers interviewed were: two social workers (SW), two nursery nurses (NN), one special educational needs (SEN) coordinator, three midwives (MW), two librarians (L), one community paediatrician (CP), one clinical psychologist (CPsy), three health visitors (HV), two speech and language therapists (S&LT), and one children's resource worker (CRW).

A purposive sampling method was used (Patton 1990). Only individuals who had made referrals to, or had received referrals from, one particular Nottinghamshire Sure Start were approached. The aim was to include a broad range of professional groups, but no attempt was made to select a random sample. In total, 20 providers were approached. None declined to be interviewed. However, two were unavailable for interview during the time-span of the project.

The interview schedule was designed following discussions with the Sure Start programme director. It was then piloted with a local social worker and refined on the basis of the pilot. All interviewees gave informed consent to be interviewed. Interviews lasted between 40 minutes and one hour and took place at a time and location suitable for the interviewee. All interviews were recorded and transcribed. Analysis was inductive and carried out manually.

Findings

All the mainstream statutory providers (hereafter referred to as mainstream providers) viewed Sure Start as a positive addition to service provision. The perception that it is a well resourced initiative was highly valued, especially in the context of mainstream provision that is perceived to be under-resourced (Edgley and Avis 2006, 2007).

Targeting provision and a 'poverty perspective'

Where mainstream providers most consistently expressed difficulty in working with Sure Start was in respect of their boundaries for targeting. Mainstream statutory providers work on a case-by-case needs basis. Sure Start's strategy of targeting resources on a particular neighbourhood by contrast produced a number of contradictions for mainstream providers. First, there were practical difficulties expressed, associated with not knowing whether their client was eligible for Sure Start provision or not. Mainstream providers worked in geographical patches, which in some cases involved three different Sure Starts, as well as an area without Sure Start provision. Not only did this mean the possibility of three different referral systems, but it also meant uncertainty about whether a client had eligibility or not.

> My biggest problem is not knowing who falls within the right catchment. (CPsy)

> It's quite confusing working with three different Sure Starts because they all have their different referral systems and information giving systems. (HV 3)

Second, there were ethical concerns produced by the anomalies of a system apparently targeted to the most deprived families, but actually determined by geographical boundary. So respondents spoke of those families recognised as 'in need' but who fell outside the boundaries of eligibility. Conversely concerns were expressed about families not deemed to be 'in need' yet able to access Sure Start services. This would either be because the Sure Start provision was offered in a public place such as a library, or because, simply by dint of having an address in a Sure Start area, families were eligible for services such as safety gates.

> We often had families that lived just across the road…we felt they were very vulnerable and they were excluded just because they lived on…the opposite side of the road. (CRW)

> because I find that people that use the groups are the people that are motivated and not necessarily in poverty. You know I've got a cluster of houses that are in the Sure Start area that are pretty middle class really. (HV 2)

A third way in which the policy of targeting resources was a concern to this particular Sure Start lay in the decision to offer the children of some parents and carers a 16-week nursery place. For many mainstream providers, while this was recognised as an extremely valuable resource, it nevertheless privileged 'acute need' rather than 'chronic need'. For many mainstream providers the problems of poverty are more likely to produce 'needs' that are chronic rather than acute.

> The mother had severe postnatal depression. It doesn't go in four months… taking that away is really, really hard after 16 weeks because sometimes the crisis doesn't go in sixteen weeks and sometimes it's not a volcano type crisis that will erupt and settle down. (HV 3)

Relatedly, some concern was also expressed that having services targeted on the basis of deprivation has the effect of undermining a professional's integrity for determining need, because deprivation is not the only determining factor in 'need'.

> Why have you got a panel? If you're working alongside a professional health visitor who truly says I need this place for this lady. Excuse me who are they to say whether that's right or wrong, if there's a space let's use it? (HV 3)

The government's agenda to 'mainstream' Sure Start services, by extending integrated service provision into Children's Centres, would presumably address many of these concerns. However, the notion that Sure Start's 'poverty perspective' should permeate and adapt mainstream service provision was also problematic for many mainstream professionals. For many the fact that Sure Start was able to offer a variety of services that statutory services could not was due to the fact that insufficient resources meant they were 'forced' to interpret their own agendas and remit fairly narrowly. This meant that they were only able to offer the statutory minimum obligations.

> So they've been keeping their head above water…everything that was there that we could've done, we'd love to have done, but we just haven't been able to. (MW 2).

Indeed the suggestion that Sure Start might have fostered innovative working practices was generally dismissed.

> A lot of the services that Sure Start actually offer they…did at the previous family centres or the day nurseries as they were before that…it's not all new stuff…some of the community ideas…we used to run toy library and book libraries…it wasn't anything really new. (CRW)

As one midwife (MW 1) put it, when comparing her job in a middle class area with her job in the Sure Start area, it was working with impoverished families that had influenced her work practices, not her contact with Sure Start.

> It was like a new kind of midwifery to me, the actual…hands on midwifery is such a small part of a much, much bigger picture. And I go home sometimes and I think I'm a housing worker, social worker, you know charity worker, I do everything. (MW 1)

Integrated and multi-professional
A key focus of the Sure Start agenda was a concern to offer services focused on the needs of families with young children from a multi-professional agency. In other words the government's desire to address the need for integrated service provision was a key aim in the Sure Start project. The work with Sure Start and its multi-professional ethos, however, appeared to have had little impact on mainstream professional perceptions of their ability to collaborate. Most mainstream providers spoke at length about working alongside other professional groups, both mainstream and voluntary. Indeed, a number spoke about having to organise and coordinate services for those families living outside the Sure Start area. Having said this, being able to access a multi-professional team was regarded as beneficial by one social worker:

> Sometimes [there are] other agencies which we can…use as opposed to just using Sure Start, but obviously a multi-agency team like Sure Start is always preferable. (SW 2)

The exception to this was the librarians. They emphasised that working with Sure Start had improved communication channels and collaboration because Sure Start had raised their profile and demonstrated the relevance of their work to healthcare workers and educationalists charged with improving the health and education of deprived groups.

> I find the things with Sure Start, it's helped in a way to give us a higher profile with other professionals. So for example…very rarely would you have the Education Department trying to work with us, they don't see us as perhaps being able to achieve their objectives… Before it was a matter of if you heard something, then trying to get in… Now we're actually invited. (L 1)

> But our constant battle really is to be taken seriously with a lot of these people, because a lot of people just think that all we do is stamp books. (L 2)

It was also acknowledged by several respondents that communication was always improved between mainstream professionals and Sure Start when they shared office space.

> I just go through X a lot of the time, I don't fill the referral form in I just say "Oh X, I've got this family that I'm working with, is there any chance that Sure Start can do a visit, see what services they can offer"? (HV 1)

Placing services under one roof in Children's Centres will clearly aid communication and collaboration in the minds of mainstream providers. It was also acknowledged that a 'one-stop shop' for a range of needs would be very beneficial to users of services.

Overall it would seem that mainstream service providers already see themselves collaborating with a range of different professionals. They also seemed very open to the idea of services being offered from under one roof. For them, if 'mainstreaming' is about interprofessional collaboration, then they were supportive of this ambition. There was, however, mixed support for the use of paraprofessionals (a trained worker who is not a member of a profession but who assists a professional).

The midwives were very supportive of working alongside 'maternity support workers'. The midwives interviewed were struggling with very high caseloads because they were short-staffed. They saw the connection between the skilled midwifery role and the extra support required by some deprived families but took the view that this support could be undertaken by someone without their skill levels.

> They're idealistic things and they're slightly outside our remit really, but they are things that we do feel frustrated that women might get depressed because they haven't got anybody around. (MW 1)

> But that's something that's been taken off us you see, because Sure Start would be able to sort out the different agencies that would get them equipment and things whereas that took a lot of our time and it's not skilled work. (MW 1)

Other professionals took a more sceptical view. In clinical psychology there was a concern that nursery nurses were being seen as a cheaper alternative for addressing behaviour problems in the community, but without appropriate training.

> And that to me is a bit worrying because in aspects of clinical governance when you're talking about how you can involve best practice, start by saying you need adequately trained staff to deliver a service. What you're doing is a bit back to front, you're starting a service but not training staff to meet the need. (CPsy)

Where all respondents questioned whether it was realistic to mainstream Sure Start services was in respect of the funding that Sure Start has enjoyed. Scepticism was expressed about whether, without the funding Sure Start has attracted, it would be possible to offer the kinds of 'value-added' services characteristic of Sure Start. Concern was also expressed about funding not being 'ring-fenced' because it would not be coming directly from government but rather via councils.

> While Sure Start has got control, from my point of view, it's better because I know it'll be spent on little ones. (L 2)

Demand-led services

A central feature of Sure Start has been that its services have been targeted at a particular community, rather than at individual need. Once an area has proved its eligibility on the basis of deprivation, funding has followed. It has then been the responsibility of Sure Start to engage with the community in determining what services that community wants and needs. The mechanism for achieving this has been the Partnership Boards. These are made up of a range of stakeholders, but significantly have included service users. In other words, Partnership Boards comprise a number of parent and carer representatives from the community to ensure services are demand-led. Once services are established Sure Start can only contact a family if the family has signed an agreement. This requires midwives and health visitors to explain the family's Sure Start entitlement, and invite them to sign up.

Most mainstream providers saw the user involvement in determining Sure Start provision as positive. Many mainstream providers articulated concern that mainstream service provision was not always trusted and that social services in particular were synonymous with children being removed into care. Sure Start's approach was more likely to engender trust.

> I think it is really good to involve local people and get their views…the only time I can remember…service users being involved in anything…was in job interviews…[but] I've not heard of it for a while. (SW 1)

However, concern was expressed about this aspect of Sure Start being lost with mainstreaming.

> If it's mainstreamed then what happens to the parents on the…board and things like that because you know if it's mainstreamed it becomes a different kettle of fish doesn't it? (NN 1)

Despite the general view that involving service users in decisions about service provision was positive, there was concern that despite their involvement, events and services were still underutilised. Some mainstream providers were unsure about the extent to which Sure Start effectively operationalised a community's 'need'.

> I think you've got to be pretty middle class to engage in a music therapy class. (HV 2)

Others were concerned that there was insufficient diversity among parent representatives to ensure the required variety in service provision.

> We find…that quite a few parents don't really like going to some of the groups and especially if they've got a child with autism, you know that their behaviour is not. (SEN)

> Quite a few of the parents are depressed and they don't like being in…bigger groups… So it's good that parents get…to say what service might be nice in their area but then I think some of the parents…get sort of missed out. (SEN)

Others, however, recognised that even though an event was identified by the 'community', this in itself did not guarantee it would be well attended.

> We were having difficulty getting the parents to come into that course and yet you know it's something that's identified by the community. (L 1)

Finally the paradox faced by many professionals was raised, that what service users might want might not be the same as what they needed. Indeed, one respondent spoke about the preliminary work that needs to be done with service users to support their decision-making, such as providing them with skills to compare outcomes between the variety of possible services within a framework of limited resources.

> Well nobody would ask for clinical psychology or health visiting…people just wouldn't ask for it…they get what they want but maybe what they get isn't what they need and you don't know what you want unless you know what you can have. (CPsy)

> The timescale for doing that kind of process is very long where you have to go and work with people to get them skilled up to…actually think about options

and think about what would be helpful and what wouldn't be, and to think about what things cost and…what has the best outcome, what the evidence suggests. (CPsy)

Another concern related to a perception that each Sure Start has set itself up without reference to 'good practice' in other Sure Starts. By working with a number of different Sure Starts, mainstream providers were in a position to compare the various ways different Sure Starts had interpreted their agenda.

My main criticism of Sure Start, the way it's cropped up over the city, is that they all do their own thing… I think a lot of reinventing the wheel has gone on. (L 2)

Of course, one deprived community's needs may be very different from another deprived community's needs. However, there was a sense that some Sure Starts were more effective at interpreting their remit than others.

Another area of concern for some mainstream providers around the demand-led nature of Sure Start services was that this meant they were seen as fragmented. Particular concern was expressed about respite care being offered in the form of a nursery place without at the same time ensuring the needs of parents or carers are addressed. So parents with depression, alcohol or drug problems were seen as not being sufficiently encouraged to address their problems while they were receiving respite.

There have been times when a child may have been here [nursery] for like six months…and nothing has been done to support that parent. (NN 1)

For other mainstream providers, however, not linking resources to one another was seen as a positive feature of Sure Start.

So it's quite good because Sure Start aren't saying…you can only have one if you have the other. (SEN)

Conclusion

Between 2002 and 2004 mainstreaming pilots were carried out to consider how strategic planners could use the experience from Sure Start to adapt mainstream early years, childcare, health and family support services to make them more integrated and responsive to children's and families' needs and provide more preventative services which better met the needs of children in poverty. Of particular interest were:

- multidisciplinary training for professionals working in children's services to help establish a common approach and knowledge base among service providers
- use of paraprofessionals to supplement the work of specialised staff, for example nursery nurses trained by speech and language therapists working with children to promote language development

or employing community parents to work alongside health visitors to support new parents

- use of information technology to create more joined-up services, for example through using common databases to improve referrals between services

- combining services in existing settings, for example by bringing health and outreach workers into childcare settings to provide a more holistic range of services. (Sure Start 2006)

It is notable that the activity undertaken in the pilots did not include exploring the use of parents in governance roles characteristic of Sure Start on their Partnership Boards. It has been acknowledged that while formal governance arrangements for Children's Centres may vary between councils, the government says 'engaging parents is fully embedded in the Children's Trust approach' (National Literacy Trust 2006).

Of the three distinctive features of Sure Start – targeting, integrated multi-professional teams, and demand-led service provision – it seems from the perspective of mainstream professionals that Sure Start has made little impression. The absence of a structure for mainstream services to be demand-led means that when Sure Start services are mainstreamed, providers are unlikely to embrace this element of Sure Start's ethos, despite the fact that it was this element that was identified by all respondents as progressive and distinctive. As targeted provision at deprived families was seen as either inappropriate, ineffective or as already established, this feature of Sure Start's work is also unlikely to leave a lasting impression. Where it seems the government is placing most emphasis in respect of mainstreaming Sure Start services is the integration and development of multi-professional teams. However, here too mainstream providers are sceptical about the impact Sure Start has had on a collaborative agenda. More significant for mainstream providers are the anticipated benefits of bringing services together under one roof in Children's Centres. Overall the mainstream providers interviewed have highly valued the service provision offered by Sure Start. However, it would seem that this has had more to do with the healthy funding that Sure Start services have attracted than a distinctive Sure Start ethos for service provision.

Implications for Children's Centres

- Sure Start has been a distinctive and popular initiative amongst service providers. However, the removal of its funding makes it difficult to conceive how demand-led services and targeted provision might continue to be supported.

- Sure Start has been important in facilitating partnership working. However, this significance may well be a function of the funding that it offered rather than indicative of creating new philosophies of partnership working.

- It is anticipated that bringing services together under one roof within Children's Centres will offer benefits in enabling mainstream service providers to work closely together.

References

Department for Children, Schools and Families (2007) *Children's trusts.* www.everychildmatters.gov.uk/aims/childrenstrusts, accessed on 23 August 2007.

Department for Education and Skills (2003) *Every Child Matters – the Green Paper.* www.literacytrust.org.uk/socialinclusion/youngpeople/greenpaper.html, accessed on 23 October 2006.

Department of Health, Department for Education and Skills (2004) *National Service Framework for Children, Young People and Maternity Services (Gateway reference 3779, product codes 20293 & 40496).* London: Department of Health.

Edgley, A. and Avis, M. (2006) 'Interprofessional collaboration: Sure Start, uncertain futures.' *Journal of Interprofessional Care 20*, 4, 433–435.

Edgley, A. and Avis, M. (2007) 'The perception of statutory service providers of a local Sure Start programme: a shared agenda?' *Health and Social Care in the Community 15*, 4, 37–386.

HM Treasury (2004) *Choice for Parents, the Best Start for Children: a Ten Year Strategy for Childcare.* London: HMSO.

House of Lords (2004) *Children Bill.* www.publications.parliament.uk/pa/ld200304/ldbills/035/2004035.htm, accessed on 23 October 2004.

McLaughlin, H. (2004) 'Partnerships: panacea or pretence?' *Journal of Professional Care 18*, 2, 103–113.

National Literacy Trust (2006) 'Mainstreaming begins for Sure Start.' www.literacytrust.org.uk/database/early.html#Mainstreaming, accessed on 20 November 2006.

Patton, M.Q. (1990) *Qualitative Evaluation and Research Methods* (2nd edition). Newbury Park, CA: Sage Publications.

Sure Start (2006) 'Mainstreaming pilots.' www.surestart.gov.uk/surestartservices/settings/surestartlocalprogrammes/history/mainstreaming, accessed on 14 November 2006.

Part 3

Paths to Education and Employment

Chapter 13

Introduction to Paths to Education and Employment

Justine Schneider

Sure Start was designed to have an impact on parents as well as children. Children were to benefit from effective interventions at a young age because these would prevent later problems and promote their health, education and lifetime productivity. Parents were encouraged into employment through Sure Start, with the promise of improved quality of life for themselves and their children as well as economic benefits for the country as a whole. Part 3 of this book looks first at the longer-term impact of early education programmes, of which Sure Start is one exemplar, and then at how Sure Start Local Programmes tackled the problem of workless households.

Sure Start as an early educational intervention

Several types of 'early interventions' with children are available in the UK, including professional child-minders, day nurseries, playgroups and nursery education. Until relatively recently, almost all the evidence in favour of such interventions had been gathered in the USA. Head Start, Early Head Start (Love *et al.* 2002), the Abecedarian project (Campbell 1996; Ramey and Ramey 1998), Perry High/Scope (Schweinhart and Weikart 1997), and Chicago Parent–Child Centres (Reynolds *et al.* 2002) received global attention. In an authoritative review, Zoritch, Roberts and Oakley (2000) draw the following conclusion from this body of research:

> Day care increases children's IQ, and has beneficial effects on behavioural development and school achievement. Long-term follow up demonstrates increased employment, lower teenage pregnancy rates, higher socioeconomic status and decreased criminal behaviour. There are positive effects on mothers' education, employment and interaction with children.

However, this is qualified in several respects. Effects on fathers have not been measured, a limited number of outcomes is examined in each study, parents are involved to different degrees in the programmes, and the studies were conducted predominantly on a poor, Black population in the United States, making it difficult to generalise the findings to other cultures and socio-economic groups. In short, day care has been shown to be cost-effective for disadvantaged USA populations but there is considerable diversity between the studies cited in support of this assertion.

UK sources of evidence are therefore of particular interest in judging the likely longer-term impact of Sure Start. We have identified two relevant studies preceding the national evaluation of Sure Start itself, whose final results are still awaited. One is summarised in this section by Alissa Goodman and Barbara Sianesi (Chapter 14). It is based on an analysis of the National Child Development Study. The authors review what is known about the impact of early interventions on short-term educational performance and longer-term economic performance. They demonstrate the implications of these results for Sure Start and similar initiatives such as Children's Centres.

The second key source is the Effective Provision of Pre-School Education (EPPE) study (Sylva *et al.* 2004). The 1997–2003 stage of the ongoing EPPE study overlapped with the Sure Start Local Programmes described in this book. Six English Local Authorities (LAs) in five regions were chosen to participate in this phase of EPPE research. These were selected to cover pre-school provision in urban, suburban and rural areas and a range of ethnic diversity and social disadvantage: playgroups, local authority or voluntary day nurseries, private day nurseries and early education. The EPPE study found that pre-school benefited all children aged three to four, and that the greater benefit arose from longer exposure (greater duration over time, not more hours per week). The benefits were sustained at least up to age seven. Full-time attendance had no more impact than part time. More disadvantaged children gained significantly, especially if they attended socially mixed settings. The quality of the centre was crucial to its impact; good quality was found in all six settings but integrated 'care and education' settings and nursery schools tended to be better than average. Children made better all round progress in settings where there was an emphasis on social development as well as on educational attainment. As to the active ingredients which seemed to be driving these findings, the number of qualified teaching staff was positively associated with children's outcomes, and the quality of the home learning environment was also important. Both of these advantages seemed to be associated with having adult carers/educators who fostered 'sustained shared thinking' and 'positive questioning' (Sylva *et al.* 2004). The importance of EPPE research in shaping the approach of the Children's Centres is reflected in the attention given to the study's findings in the *Choice for Parents, the Best Start for Children: a Ten Year Strategy for Childcare* (HM Treasury 2004).

Employment

The specification of targets for the 2003–2004 to 2005–2006 Public Service Agreement (Sure Start 2002) included as its fourth objective: 'In fully operational programmes, to achieve by 2005–2006 a 12 per cent reduction in the proportion of young children (aged 0–4) living in households where no-one is working'. Although this objective was implemented in most places only after the programmes had addressed children's health, learning, social and emotional development, many programmes offered parents opportunities to improve literacy, numeracy and computer skills. In addition, participation in the local programme came to be seen as a means for parents to acquire work-related skills and experience, increasing their chances of employment and thus helping to achieve this target.

The second and third chapters in Part 3 are concerned with processes, initiated through Sure Start programmes, whereby parents moved closer to paid employment. The first looks at Sure Start as a step towards formal employment in contexts beyond the programme itself. Mairi-Ann Cullen and Geoff Lindsay (Chapter 15) describe the Chelmsley Wood local programme's adult tutor project, a model whose promising results suggest that it could usefully be developed in other settings. Matthew Pearson and Ann Martin (Chapter 16) explore the issues raised by parents' formal employment within the Askern Sure Start Local Programme and reflect on parents' involvement as providers of the same statutory services which they might have received.

References

Campbell, F.A. (1996) *The Effects of Intensive Early Childhood Educational Intervention on Assignments to Special Education in School: the Abecedarian Study*. Boston, MA: Society for Research in Adolescents.

HM Treasury (2004) *Choice for Parents, the Best Start for Children: a Ten Year Strategy for Childcare*. Norwich: HMSO.

Love, J.M., Kisker, E.E., Ross, C.M., Schochet, P.Z., *et al.* (2002) *Making a Difference in the Lives of Infants and Toddlers and their Families: The Impacts of Early Head Start*. Washington, DC: US Department of Health and Human Services.

Ramey, C.T. and Ramey, S.L. (1998) 'Early intervention and early experience.' *American Psychologist 53*, 109–120.

Reynolds, A.J., Temple, J., Robertson, D. and Mann, E. (2002) *Age 21 Cost–Benefit Analysis of the Title I Chicago Parent–Child Centers*. Madison, WI: Institute for Research on Poverty.

Schweinhart, L.J. and Weikart, D.P. (1997) 'The High/Scope preschool curriculum comparison study through age 23.' *Early Childhood Research Quarterly 12*, 2, 117–143.

Sure Start (2002) *PSA Targets 2003–2006. Technical Note for Public Service Agreement 2003–04 to 2005–06*. www.surestart.gov.uk/_doc/P000151.doc, accessed on 20 April 2007.

Sylva, K., Melhuish, E., Sammons, P., Siraj-Blatchford, I. and Taggart, B. (2004) *Effective Pre-School Education*. www.surestart.gov.uk/_doc/P0001378.pdf, accessed on 20 April 2007.

Zoritch, B., Roberts. I. and Oakley, A. (2000) 'Day care for pre-school children.' *Cochrane Database of Systematic Reviews 2000*, Issue 3. (Art. No.: CD000564. DOI: 10.1002/14651858.CD000564.)

Chapter 14

Early Education and Children's Outcomes: How Long Do the Impacts Last?

Alissa Goodman and Barbara Sianesi

Early childcare and pre-school policies have become an important focus of the government's strategy for improving children's outcomes, either through direct effects of early education on children, or through the enabling effect that childcare has on allowing parents to work. Key recent initiatives in this context are Sure Start and Children's Centres.

The aim of this chapter is to shed light on the question of how effective early schooling and pre-school are in improving the well-being of children, and whether any impacts are likely to be long-lasting. The chapter draws from Goodman and Sianesi (2006), a research paper which itself added to a well-established literature, both from the UK and from the rest of the world (especially the USA). The unique contribution of our work stems from the fact that we study the long-term effects of early education amongst a cohort that has now reached adulthood. By contrast, most existing studies have looked at early education amongst contemporary cohorts of children, and by their very nature are unable to be informative as to the longer-term effects.

Data and methodology

Data

Our work uses a sample of children from the National Child Development Study (NCDS), a longitudinal study of a single cohort of people born in Britain in 1958. We have assembled information from when cohort members were aged 0, 7, 11, 16, 23, 33, and 42. The individual data have in turn been combined with information about state-maintained provision of nursery places at the local authority (LA) level, as well as other information about LA characteristics. The sample we have chosen consists of 12,513 children with non-missing pre-school information.[1,2] The data are used to construct variables that measure the early education 'treatments', our outcomes of interest and a detailed set of control variables. We briefly discuss each of these in turn.

We estimate the effects of the following two broad types of treatments, or investments, in early education:

1. *Pre-compulsory* education encompasses *any* formal early education prior to the compulsory school starting age of five. This education can take place either in a school setting through *early school entry* (i.e. before the first autumn term after a child turns five), or in a *pre-school setting* such as state-maintained or private nursery or playgroup.

2. *Nursery or playgroup attendance* is restricted to early learning only in a *pre-school setting*, which includes state-maintained and private nurseries as well as playgroups.

Whilst the former treatment allows us to answer the question of whether any education before the age of five has any short- or long-term effects, the latter addresses the question of whether attendance at nursery or playgroups before entering primary school has any short- or long-term effects. This second treatment definition reflects more closely the provision of Sure Start Children's Centres for children under five living in the most disadvantaged areas.[3]

In the following, when there is no need to distinguish between the two types of treatment, we will use the encompassing term of *early education*.

We consider a wide range of children's outcomes, from cognitive development, as measured by a series of tests taken at ages 7, 11 and 16, to socialisation, derived from both parental and teacher assessments of social skills also at 7, 11 and 16, as well as educational attainment and labour market outcomes up to the age of 42. The measures we use are summarised in Table 14.1.

As we describe in some more detail below, our estimation strategy relies on the quality of the control variables we can use to adjust for selective differences between children who participated in early education and those who did not. The wide-ranging set of characteristics of the child, the parents, the home-learning environment and the local area are summarised in Table 14.2.

Table 14.1 Selected outcomes

Outcome	Our measure
Cognitive development	
Overall cognitive development at 7	Average score over all tests[a] (std)
Mathematical skills at 7	Problem Arithmetic Test score (std)
Reading skills at 7	Southgate Group Reading Test score (std)
Overall cognitive development at 11	Average score over all tests[a] (std)
Mathematical skills at 11	Mathematics test score (std)
Reading skills at 11	Reading comprehension test score (std)
Overall cognitive development at 16	Average score over both tests[a] (std)
Mathematical skills at 16	Mathematics test score (std)
Reading skills at 16	Reading comprehension test score (std)
Social/behavioural development	
Overall social development at 7	*Teacher*: BSAG total score of behaviour deviance[b] (std)
Very bad 'interpersonal' skills at 7	*Parent*: Proportion of very bad interpersonal skills out of: over-depends on mother (teacher-assessed), meets other kids outside household; fights other children; bullied by other kids and disobedient
Very bad 'self-control' skills at 7	*Parent*: Proportion of very bad self-control skills out of: generally destructive; irritable; difficulty concentrating; upset by new situation; miserable or tearful and has temper tantrums
Overall social development at 11	*Teacher*: BSAG total score of behaviour deviance[b] (std)
Offending behaviour at 11	*Teacher*: Pre-delinquent, rebellious, aggressive

Continued on next page

Table 14.1 *cont.*

Outcome	Our measure
Very bad social skills at 11	*Parent*: Proportion of very bad skills out of: difficulty settling to anything; destroys own/others' things; irritable; upset by new situation; fights with other children; bullied by other children; disobedient at home and miserable or tearful
Overall teacher social assessment at 16	Proportion of very bad skills out of 13
Overall parental social assessment at 16	Proportion of very bad skills out of 12
Offending behaviour at 16	*Parent*: Has had trouble with the police or been to court
Educational attainment	
Special education at 7	Helped/would need help for backwardness/special school
Any qualification	Has obtained any qualification above Level 1 by age 42
Higher education	Has obtained any qualification at Level 4 or 5 by age 42
Labour market success	
Employment status at 33 and 42	Employee or self-employed
Wages at 33 and 42	Real hourly gross pay (log)

(std): standardised to mean zero and unit variance

[a] Average over all tests administered at that age. More than maths and reading tests make up the average for ages 7 and 11. At all ages, the average score is calculated based on any available test score; sample sizes might thus differ

[b] The *Bristol Social Adjustment Guide* (BSAG) is intended to detect and classify behaviour (social adjustment) disturbances in school-age-children. Designed to be as free as possible from the unreliability of personal judgement, it is completed by a teacher who has observed the child's behaviour

Table 14.2 Summary of control variables

Child

Characteristics	*Early development*
Gender	Handicaps
Ethnicity	Attended welfare clinic under 1 year
Mother's usual language with child is not English	Not walking alone by 1.5 years
	Not speaking by 2 years
Birth weight	Incontinent by day after 3 years
Illness noted at birth	
Breastfed	

Parents

Pregnancy history

Past miscarriages, neonatal deaths or complications

Interval between marriage and first birth

Human capital

Father's years of education

Mother's years of education

Mother reads newspaper most days and books most weeks

Father reads newspaper most days and books most weeks

Socioeconomic status

Maternal grandfather's social class

Paternal grandfather's social class

Social class of mother's husband

Health/demographics

Mother's age

Father's age

Mother's intensity of smoking prior to pregnancy

Stopped smoking in pregnancy

Mother is obese

UK region where mother was born

Mother's labour supply at pregnancy

Social class (type of paid job)

Works over 40 hours in pregnancy

Stops work after 29 weeks in pregnancy

Continued on next page

Table 14.2 *cont.*

Home / learning environment

Family type
Mother's marital status at birth: married, unmarried or separated, divorced or widowed

Child in care by age 7

Family difficulties
Physical illness or disability

Mental illness, neurosis or subnormality

Divorce, separation, desertion; domestic/in-law tension

Alcoholism

Other serious difficulties

Parental time
Child has twin

Birth order

Any older brother

Any older sister

Has close sibling

Family size

Local characteristics

Administrative County or County Borough

Region

LA demographic composition ('65)
Primary students/1000 population

Secondary students/1000 population

LA local income/employment structure ('61)
Active females as % of active males

% males in semi- and unskilled occupations

Relative weight given by LA to nursery ('58)
Nursery pupils as % of total pupils

Nursery pupils per teacher over all pupils per teacher

Quality of primary, secondary education in LA ('65)
Primary teachers' salary – cost per pupil

Secondary teachers' salary – cost per pupil

All primary school costs per pupil

All secondary school costs per pupil

Methodology

We are interested in the causal effect of early education – either in the form of pre-compulsory education or attendance at nursery/playgroups – on the cognitive and behavioural development of those children attending early education. Note also that we are concerned with the *total* effect of early education on achievement, that is, not holding other family and school inputs constant. Such effects thus also encompass the indirect contribution of any other concurrent and subsequent family and school inputs that change as a result of participation in early education and in turn affect cognitive development.[4]

In this chapter we present estimates of these effects based on standard ordinary least squares (OLS) regression. This method allows us to control for any observable characteristic that determines both whether or not a child participates in early education as well as the child's subsequent outcomes. Since children who attend early education are not likely to be a random subsample of the overall child population (the 'selection-bias' problem), the validity of the regression approach rests primarily on the assumption that we can observe all the relevant characteristics that determine participation in early education. We argue in some detail in our main paper (Goodman and Sianesi 2006) that a case can indeed be made that we can capture in the NCDS data all the relevant child characteristics, family background influences, parental inputs and local characteristics upon which parents are likely to take their early education decisions (c.f. Table 14.2). However, it should be noted that even if all the characteristics determining selection into early education were observable to researchers, OLS may still suffer from some potential sources of bias.[5] In our more extensive work we have investigated the robustness of our OLS estimates by comparing them to effects estimated using other methodologies, including propensity score matching and fully interacted regression models (for a discussion of these two methods see for example Blundell, Dearden and Sianesi 2005). We found that in general OLS performed very well against these other estimation techniques and therefore we present only our OLS estimates here.

Results

Background

Tables 14.3 and 14.4 show the patterns of participation in early education for children born in 1958. As many as 60 per cent of these children had some form of schooling prior to the statutory school starting age of five (Table 14.3). For the large majority (three-quarters) this early education was only in terms of an early start to infant school. A considerable number, however, attended a pre-school placement, with roughly an equal share (over 10%) being in the maintained and private sectors. In the latter group, an almost equal proportion (5–6%) started their early education in a nursery as in the less formal setting of playgroups.

If by contrast we focus strictly on attendance at nursery/playgroups without taking into account whether the child subsequently started school early, the picture changes markedly (Table 14.4). Around 15 per cent of the children attended a nursery or playgroup, a considerably smaller share than the 60 per cent who received *any* early education, as most of the latter were early school entrants. Again we see an equal split between maintained and independent institutions and, within the latter, between nurseries and playgroups.

Table 14.3 Sample split by type of pre-compulsory education

	Number	%
No pre-compulsory education	4343	39.7
Any pre-compulsory education	6605	60.3
of whom:		
– Only entered school early	4921	74.5
– LEA nursery[a]	831	12.6
– Private nursery[a]	371	5.6
– Playgroup (62% also with early schooling)	377	5.7
– Nursery and playgroup[a]	105	1.6

[a] Some also with early schooling

Table 14.4 Sample split by type of pre-school (nursery or playgroup) education

	Number	%
No pre-school education (53.1% of whom entered school early)	9266	84.6
Any pre-school education	1684	15.4
of whom:		
– LEA nursery[a]	831	49.3
– Private nursery[a]	371	22.0
– Playgroup (62% also with early schooling)	377	22.4
– Nursery and playgroup[a]	105	6.2

[a] Some also with early schooling

The average personal, parental, home environment and regional characteristics of the children receiving early education differed in important ways from those of children with no early education experience. In particular, a child who was underprivileged for social or economic reasons (proxied by social class) was shown to be far *less* likely to have had any experience of nursery/playgroup or to have started school early than a relatively more advantaged child. These disparities are likely to be further compounded by the large differences we found in the availability and experience of nurseries, playgroups and early school entry, depending on the social, demographic and economic profiles of the regions and LAs they lived in.[6]

The effects of pre-compulsory education

Of particular interest is the effect of pre-compulsory education on cognitive development. The first column of Table 14.5 shows our OLS estimates of the effects of pre-compulsory education on a range of standardised test scores taken between age 7 and 16 accounting for variation in the factors listed in Table 14.2. The results confirm that pre-compulsory education leads to consistently better test scores, both on average, and separately in maths and reading, at age seven. Importantly, we also find that these gains persist, though diminished in size, through to ages 11 and 16. In particular, the results suggest that obtaining education before the age of five is associated with an increase of nine per cent of a standard deviation in average test scores at age seven; by age 11, the gain is around seven per cent; by age 16 this has declined to just over half its size at age seven, but remains highly statistically significant at around five per cent.

How economically significant are these effects? Table 14.5 shows that whilst the positive effects of pre-compulsory education on test scores are larger than the effect of having a father with a high social class at age seven, the advantage conferred by social class is magnified over time, whilst the effects of pre-compulsory education diminish. Similarly, whilst the positive effect of pre-compulsory education is of approximately the same magnitude (but opposite direction) as the detrimental effects associated with living in a family with severe difficulties at age seven, the effects of the family difficulties persist basically unchanged over time, whilst the effects of pre-compulsory education are greatly diminished.

The picture of how pre-compulsory education affects social skills is more mixed than the picture for cognitive skills. Table 14.5 shows that education before age five leads to better teacher-reported social skills but to some worse parental reports at age seven. Further, while the positive early effect on teacher-reported behavioural adjustment does not appear to be long-lasting, the increased negative perception by parents persists until age 11. By contrast, markedly large, negative effects on socialisation from a difficult home

Table 14.5 Effects of pre-school compulsory education on measures of cognition and socialisation, and coefficients on other aspects of the home environment (OLS estimates)

		Pre-compulsory education	Father's social class I or II	Difficult home environment	Mother's years of education
Cognition					
at 7	Average	0.090***	0.055***	−0.096***	0.024***
	Maths	0.141***	0.098***	−0.191***	0.044***
	Reading	0.165***	0.102***	−0.264***	0.033***
at 11	Average	0.067***	0.135***	−0.086***	0.032***
	Maths	0.119***	0.255***	−0.221***	0.051***
	Reading	0.084***	0.203***	−0.152***	0.058***
at 16	Average	0.048***	0.091**	−0.090***	0.029***
	Maths	0.069***	0.243***	−0.189***	0.062***
	Reading	0.071***	0.148***	−0.184***	0.040***
Socialisation					
at 7	BSAG[a] (T)	−0.053***	−0.058**	0.205***	−0.007
	Very bad interpersonal skills (P)	0.002	−0.008***	0.028***	0.000
	Very bad self-control skills (P)	0.008***	−0.014***	0.032***	−0.001
at 11	BSAG[a] (T)	−0.018	−0.041	0.233***	−0.018*
	Very bad social skills (P)	0.006**	−0.008***	0.021***	−0.002*
	Pre/Delinquent (T)	0.002	−0.005	0.018***	−0.000
at 16	Police trouble / to court	0.005	−0.013	0.062***	−0.002

*** Significant at 1%, ** at 5%, * at 10%
(T): teacher's report
(P): parental report
[a] total standardised score of behavioural *mal*adjustment
See Table 14.1 for detailed definitions

environment are found across all ages. To a lesser extent, high paternal social class is linked to positive social development at the early age and parental view of socialisation at 11, while for this 1958 cohort of children, additional years of mother's education had only a small impact at the later age.

In terms of educational outcomes, pre-compulsory education is found to have positive effects on the lower end only. In particular, early education is linked to a four percentage points lower probability of needing special education and to a three percentage points higher likelihood of obtaining some qualifications at Level 1 or above. However, we could not detect any impact on the probability of obtaining higher education qualifications. We also detected some fairly weak statistical evidence of positive labour market effects, with pre-compulsory schooling exerting a marginally significant positive effect on the probability of being in employment at age 33 (less than two percentage points gain, significant only at the 10% level) and on wages at age 33 (a 2.7% gain, again significant only at the 10% level).[7] By age 42, however, any effect has disappeared.

The effects of nursery or playgroup attendance

The next effects we consider are those of receiving pre-school education, summarised in Table 14.6. Nursery or playgroup attendance leads to higher average test scores at age seven, driven in particular by a better performance in maths. This evidence of positive effects on early cognitive performance is consistent with the findings from the EPPE study, which considers the effects of pre-school education on cognitive tests up to age seven for a cohort of today's young children (Sammons *et al.* 2004). But in contrast to pre-compulsory education more generally, we find only weak, and somewhat mixed, evidence of any long-lasting effects on cognitive scores.

As to social skills, we do not find any evidence of an improvement in teacher reports for those attending nurseries or playgroups. Parental reports of the incidence of poor skills, particularly those related to aspects of self-control of the child, are however significantly higher at age seven if the child attended pre-school. This negative effect persists up to age 11, but not to age 16.

There do not seem to be any long-lasting effects of attending nurseries or playgroups on education and labour market outcomes, the only exception being a marginally significant positive effect of 3.6 per cent on wages at age 33. This is consistent with the lack of persistence of effects on cognition and other skills, which are known to contribute to academic achievement and labour market success.

Conclusions

Our research has found that investments in human capital before the age of five appear to have had long-lasting and positive effects on the children from the

Table 14.6 Effects of attending a nursery and/or playgroup on measures of cognition and socialisation (OLS estimates)

Cognitive test scores			*Socialisation*		
at 7	Average	0.053***	at 7	BSAG[a]	0.024
	Maths	0.083***		Very bad interpersonal skills	0.003
	Reading	0.028		Very bad self-control skills	0.014***
at 11	Average	0.036**	at 11	BSAG[a]	0.040
	Maths	0.024		Very bad social skills	0.010***
	Reading	0.044*		Pre/delinquent	0.008
at 16	Average	0.005	at 16	Police trouble/to court	0.013
	Maths	0.051*			
	Reading	−0.007			

*** Significant at 1%, ** at 5%, * at 10%
(T): teacher's report
(P): parental report
[a] total standardised score of behavioural *mal*adjustment
See Table 14.1 for detailed definitions.

1958 cohort. Pre-compulsory education was found to lead to improvements in cognitive tests, diminishing in size but remaining significant throughout the schooling years up to age 16. The effects on socialisation appear to be more mixed, but are not long-lasting. We have also presented evidence that there are gains from pre-compulsory education in adulthood, in terms of a higher probability of obtaining qualifications, and in turn marginally higher employment probabilities and wages at age 33.

Our research has also shown that there is a positive impact on early test scores of attending nurseries or playgroups before a young person starts primary education. However, these effects are found to be smaller and shorter lasting than those from pre-compulsory education, with only very weak evidence of continued effects through to age 16. Similarly, we find evidence of adverse behavioural effects from parental reports at age seven, persisting to age 11, but no longer detectable by age 16.

Even though our results pertain to the early education experiences of children born in 1958, our findings are broadly in line with those for the 1970 birth cohort (Osborn and Milbank 1987), as well as those for the more recent EPPE study (Sammons *et al.* 2004). Although we cannot determine how representative of current provision the early learning experience of the NCDS children was, it is likely that any intervening changes in the practice, curriculum and organisation would have worked towards increasing the quality of the educational experience provided. Thus the long-term benefits of pre-compulsory education uncovered for the 1958 cohort are plausibly going to be even larger for current children.

Although our findings failed to identify significant long-term effects of attending nurseries or playgroups (as opposed to starting school early), our work nevertheless underlines the role that the Sure Start initiative might play in improving early cognitive performance for children in relatively disadvantaged areas by making available good quality pre-school education. Despite the fact that early findings from the National Evaluation of Sure Start were mixed (NESS Research Team 2005) they pertain to the experience of children who were at most three years old. It would in fact seem important also to assess the impact of Sure Start on less immediate outcomes, such as school performance and later educational attainment. This will be an important focus for future evaluation of Children's Centres and similar initiatives.

Implications for Children's Centres

- High quality educational environments for pre-school children should be fundamental to local provision.

- Consideration should be given to prioritising children with problems at home in allocating pre-school educational opportunities, which compensate partly for such disadvantage.

- The impact of Children's Centres needs to be measured over time, monitoring children's performance at school and even to adulthood.

Notes

1   This chapter is based on research funded by Her Majesty's Treasury Evidence Based Policy Fund in conjunction with the Department for Education and Skills, the Department of Work and Pension, Her Majesty's Customs and Excise, and the Department of Media, Culture and Sport, to whom we are very grateful. We also gratefully acknowledge co-funding from the ESRC through the Centre for the Microeconomic Analysis of Public Policy at IFS. The usual disclaimer applies.

2   We have further excluded children: (a) not present in the birth survey; (b) living in Scotland (the Scottish school system differs in a number of respects from the English one – besides, LA information was not available for Scotland); or (c) attending day nurseries (the primary aim of which was the care and protection of young vulnerable children rather than education – furthermore, less than three per cent of the NCDS children attended them).

3   Note, though, that in addition to early learning, this programme offers a host of child and family health and support services which go well beyond our definition of 'nursery and playgroups'.

4   For example, mothers of children at nursery may be induced to go back to work and thus generate more financial resources but also change the amount (and possibly quality) of time they spend with their child. All these indirect effects would be captured in our estimates.

5   First, if the true model were non-linear in the characteristics, the OLS estimate would in general be biased. Second, this regression constrains the impact to be the same for all children; if, by contrast, the effect varies according to some of the child's characteristics, OLS will not in general recover the parameter of interest. Both these biases are exacerbated if there are children participating in early education for whom there are no comparable children in the non-participating sample. In this case, performing OLS might hide the fact that the researcher is actually comparing incomparable children by using the (linear) extrapolation.

6   These inequalities were one motive for the targeting of Sure Start at more disadvantaged areas from the outset.

7   Wage effects need in general to be interpreted with caution due to potential differential selection into employment, especially given the presence of a small effect on employment probability.

References

Blundell, R., Dearden, L. and Sianesi, B. (2005) 'Evaluating the effect of education on earnings: models, methods and results from the National Child Development Survey.' *Journal of the Royal Statistical Society, Series A 168*, 3, 473–512.

Goodman, A. and Sianesi, B. (2006) 'Early education and children's outcomes: how long do the impacts last?' *Fiscal Studies 26*, 4, 513–548.

NESS Research Team (2005) *Early Impacts of Sure Start Local Programmes on Children and Families.* National Evaluation Report No. 13. www.ness.bbk.ac.uk/documents activities/impact/1183.pdf, accessed on 20 April 2007.

Osborn, A.F. and Milbank, J.E. (1987) *The Effects of Early Education: A Report from the Child Health and Education Study.* Oxford: Clarendon Press.

Sammons, P., Sylva, K., Melhuish, E.C., Siraj-Blatchford, I., Taggart, B., Elliot, K. and Marsh, A. (2004) 'The Effective Provision of Pre-School Education (EPPE) Project.' *Technical Paper 11 – The Continuing Effects of Pre-school Education at Age 7 Years.* London: DfES and Institute of Education, University of London.

Chapter 15

Lifelong Learning and Parental Employability

Mairi-Ann Cullen and Geoff Lindsay

This chapter addresses the Sure Start experience of promoting the employability of parents of children under four years of age. It begins by setting the context for a policy focus on parental employability. The second section describes a typology of approaches adopted in Sure Start Local Programmes (SSLPs) to improve parental employability and the evidence to support a lifelong learning approach. The predominantly lifelong learning approach adopted in one case study local programme is then described in detail, including evidence of the impact of this approach. The chapter concludes by drawing out lessons for Children's Centres across England.

The policy context for a target to increase parental employability

Since 1997, the government's stated aim has been to achieve both a strong economy and greater social justice (Labour Party 2005). A key focus has been 'improving the life chances of children and young people and delivering equality of opportunity' with the rationale that such support 'is an investment in a skilled and productive workforce and a more cohesive society in the future' (HM Treasury and Department for Education and Skills, 2005, p.3). This focus illustrates Levitas' analysis (2004) that New Labour policy has reflected a belief in labour market participation as the best route to social inclusion.

The policy focus on improving life chances for children and young people is important because comparative evidence showed that, by the mid 1990s and until 2000, the United Kingdom had the highest child poverty rate in the European Union (EU) (Bradshaw 2006). In 1999, therefore, the government committed to halving child poverty by 2010–2011, from 1998–1999 rates, and to eradicating it by 2020. For the purposes of monitoring, poverty was defined as a household income 60 per cent or less of the median in that year. In 2003, a more nuanced approach to defining child poverty was adopted which took into account absolute low income, relative low income and material deprivation (HM Treasury and Department for Education and Skills 2005).

The introduction of SSLPs in the most disadvantaged areas of England was one mechanism designed to tackle child poverty. Under the national objective of 'Strengthening Families and Communities', SSLPs had a target of reducing by at least 12 per cent the number of nought- to three-year-old children living in households where no-one was working by 2005–2006 (HM Treasury 2000). The target reflected the fact that the proportion of children living in workless households had increased by almost three times between the mid 1970s and mid 1990s (HM Treasury and Department for Education and Skills 2005). Also, compared to other EU countries, the UK had the highest proportion of children living in workless households and the highest proportion of children living with unemployed lone parents (Ritakallio and Bradshaw 2006). But the link between parental unemployment and child poverty is not direct; it is mediated by government policies relating to welfare benefits, wages and taxation (Bradshaw 2006; Pantazis, Gordon and Levitas 2006). In the UK, although the child benefit package has improved since 2001, it has been shown to be 'less effective in reducing poverty than it might otherwise be' (Bradshaw 2006, p.11). The Sure Start target to reduce the number of workless households reflected a specific policy choice to tackle child/family poverty through promoting parental employment rather than by addressing structural inequalities through redistribution of wealth (Levitas 2004). Given this policy approach, it was important that SSLPs adopted effective ways of supporting parents into work.

A typology of SSLP approaches to promoting parental employability

Defining employability as 'the capacity to gain and keep a job, to cope with changes at work and in the wider economy, and the ability to get a new job if necessary' (p.2), Meadows and Garbers (2004) identified five types of SSLP approaches to improving parental employability. They described these as:

- *active* approaches: collaborating with a range of agencies; positive encouragement for parents to take advantage of opportunities offered; identification of obstacles and help in overcoming these; strong links with employment and training agencies

- *lifelong learning* approaches: responsive to parents' expressed wishes for education and training; encouragement to return to learning; supportive of progression from basic to advanced training provided by other agencies; strong links with education and training programmes; emphasis on skill development rather than immediate employment; less well developed links with agencies delivering employment support

- *intermediate labour market* approaches: structuring job opportunities, recruitment and training within the SSLP to enable employment of local people; providing work experience and job related training to local parents

- *passive* approaches: offering access to mainstream employment and training provision (but not offering any extra encouragement, support or help)

- *disengaged* approaches: limited links with other agencies; no active encouragement to parents to improve employability; little or no provision of services relevant to employability.

Evidence to support effectiveness of a lifelong learning approach

As Gallie (2004a) notes, effective policies to get people back to work need to be based on evidence about the barriers that prevent people from re-entering the labour market. What evidence is there to indicate that one SSLP approach might have been better than another in increasing parental employability? Comparative evidence from EU-funded international studies shows that skill deficiencies are the biggest risk factor associated with unemployment (Gallie 2004b). Gallie (2004a) argues that, 'The quality of policy responses [to unemployment] must be judged ultimately in terms of how far they help to raise the initial skills and provide a mechanism for the renewal of skills across people's working lives' (p.31).

There is now a wealth of national and comparative research that supports the argument that a lifelong learning approach, appropriately complemented by active and intermediate labour market approaches, is an effective way of improving parental employability. For example, a systematic review (Dench, Hillage and Coare 2006) noted the effectiveness, in relation to employment outcomes for unemployed, low qualified adults, of learning being provided alongside individual, integrated support, such as help with job searching, financial and personal issues. Both Jenkins *et al.* (2003) and Conlon (2005) have shown that adult education and training have a positive impact on the chances of gaining and retaining a job.

McIntosh (2004) also argues that, 'The policy prescription to prevent high unemployment and inactivity rates, and hence social exclusion amongst those left behind with low-level skills, must be to continue to increase the skills they hold' (p.163) and that, 'Learning must be provided and supported throughout life' (p.164). This whole body of research into 'the underlying sources of labour market vulnerability and the barriers that prevent people from re-entering employment' (Gallie 2004b, p.1) provides strong evidence that a lifelong learning approach is effective in improving parents' employability.

The case of Sure Start Chelmsley Wood

In its bid for SSLP status (NCH Action for Children 2001), the Sure Start Chelmsley Wood partnership indicated the adoption of a lifelong learning approach to improving parental employability. An adult tutor role was envisaged in the context of addressing the target to reduce the number of children aged birth to three years living in workless households. This reflected the local programme's view that the tension between, on the one hand, parents' wishes to care for their own young children and, on the other hand, the government's desire to address child poverty by encouraging parents (including lone parents) of young children to take up paid employment, could best be resolved by supporting parents to be 'skilled up to return to work when ready', as one interviewee put it (Cullen and Lindsay 2005).

This tension between 'encouraging parents to go out to work and supporting the belief of many parents that part of being a good parent is to be at home with children when they are young' was also noted by Meadows and Garbers (2004, p.3). This belief about 'good parents' is not limited to disadvantaged Sure Start areas (see, for example, Barnes *et al.* 2006; Jenkins 2006). Nor is this belief in the importance of full-time parental care of young children limited to England (see, for example, van Wels and Knijn 2006). Research also suggests that it is not clear cut that working parents, particularly working mothers, are an unequivocal good (see, for example, Nomaguchi and Milkie 2006). Meadows and Garbers argued that the range of SSLP approaches to promoting parental employability, from active to disengaged, partly reflected this tension over whether young children's best interests were served (a) by being cared for by a parent (usually the mother), or (b) by parents (including lone parents) being encouraged to find paid employment to raise the family income and protect the child/ren from living in poverty.

In Sure Start Chelmsley Wood, the adult tutor role was taken on by a full-time experienced tutor seconded from the local further education (FE) college. Embedded in the SSLP, she liaised with other college tutors to ensure the provision of training and education to meet the needs and requests of parents. The college had prior successful experience of supporting work-based learning through an adult tutor seconded to a local industry. 'It has worked well to have someone employed by the college but embedded in the institution because people see them around and see them as non-threatening. I've used that model with industry, too' (college staff interviewee). The adult tutor signposted parents to learning and employment opportunities but also worked with them to address barriers to learning so that they could gain the skills to enter or re-enter the labour market when they so wished. The role included a number of elements:

- one-to-one work with parent members
- a training role with the Sure Start team and with parents

- liaison with the local FE college around provision of Family Learning courses at the Sure Start Centre and of other local adult education

- liaison at local authority level to influence lifelong learning strategy.

Main approach adopted to enhance parental employability

The main method of supporting parents to return to education, training and/or employment was a lifelong learning approach based on one-to-one work using 'learning conversations' underpinned by the 'Solihull Approach'. Learning conversations are an educational strategy based on social learning theory, as developed by Harri-Augstein and Thomas (1991). The Solihull Approach (Douglas 1999; Douglas and Brennan 2004) is a brief intervention model designed for professionals working with families, which integrates three concepts drawn from separate disciplines: containment from psychoanalytical theory, reciprocity from child development theory, and behaviour management from behaviourism.

The adult tutor described her use of learning conversations as being designed 'to encourage students to become self-organised learners' by:

> Getting them to work out what the problem is, strategies to overcome it, what will be the outcome if they use these strategies and how will they know when they've arrived at where they want to be. It's getting them to think it through, but building on their *strengths* rather than what they can't do.

Whilst acknowledging that this approach took time 'especially for students that have a lot of barriers', the benefit for the parent/learner was seen as a sense of agency and empowerment.

Learning conversations were viewed as coherent with the Solihull Approach used by all staff across the local programme. From the adult tutor's perspective, the most relevant aspect of the Solihull Approach for her role was the concept of containment, which she described in relation to adults as 'making them feel OK, making them feel very comfortable and connected with you' and enabling them 'to feel you've got space in your head for them'. Establishing this rapport, in her view, required having respect for people, spending time listening carefully, establishing two-way communication, not jumping to immediate judgements about any given situation, being alert for cues that issues other than the spoken one could be involved, not offering solutions, being prepared to signpost to other professionals.

The 'lifelong learning plus' approach

Meadows and Garbers (2004) made two criticisms of the lifelong learning approach to improving parental employability. They argued that it emphasised skill development rather than immediate employment and that it created weak links with agencies delivering employment support compared to those offering education and training. In Sure Start Chelmsley Wood, these were countered by the main lifelong learning approach being complemented by additional activity falling under the *active* and *intermediate labour market* approaches, creating a 'lifelong learning plus' approach.

Regarding an *active* approach to promoting employability, Sure Start Chelmsley Wood's adult tutor role covered all four aspects described by Meadows and Garbers (2004). In terms of collaborating with a range of local agencies, she instigated a Family Learning Network which brought together key operational-level people (from Sure Start, the FE college, the local council and local library) who were then able to plan and advertise Family Learning and to promote the national Skills for Life agenda in a coordinated and mutually supportive way. The vision was that all those working with families would be able to access training, such as the Step into Learning training and development programme, which teaches participants to recognise adults' learning needs and how to engage them in learning, and that Family Learning courses would be offered in all local Early Years settings. The adult tutor also joined relevant local strategic-level committees. She explained that this enabled her to 'feed back the voice of the learner... I see that as fitting in with the whole Sure Start ethos about sustainability and tailoring services for the needs of the community'.

Encouraging parents to take advantage of opportunities offered around employability was achieved through one-to-one learning conversations but also through information stands and signposting to other sources of support. Strong links with employment and training agencies were made primarily through the Jobcentre Plus, whose advisers, including Lone Parent Advisers, kept up-to-date information on display in the Sure Start Centre and were a regular presence there. Staff in both places ensured that parents accessing either, who would also benefit from the other, were signposted to that support. Identifying obstacles to employability and helping parents to overcome these was a key part of the learning conversations' work.

In terms of an *intermediate labour market* approach to promoting parental employability, the adult tutor had a training role which included training parents to take up a range of roles as volunteers across the programme, thus gaining work-related skills, and working with parent representatives on the Partnership Board to enable them to play a full part on the Board alongside professionals. Sure Start Chelmsley Wood also included parents on every panel interviewing applicants for jobs on the local programme and encouraged local parents to apply. As a result, by 2004, 30 of 33 volunteers were local programme area parents, as were three full-time team members and eight of 18 part-time workers (the other ten were parents who lived just outside the local programme area).

Case studies of parents' journeys to employability

In a guide (Sure Start Unit and Daycare Trust 2004) to help local programmes support parents into paid work the process involved was conceptualised as having four steps: building confidence, accessing childcare, developing new skills and helping parents apply for paid work. Analysis of the journeys made by eight case study mothers in Sure Start Chelmsley Wood (Cullen and Lindsay 2005) suggested, however, that a number of smaller steps need to be accounted for in any such conceptualisation of the journey to employability.

The steps taken by these mothers were: finding out about the SSLP; deciding to engage with it; using the Sure Start Centre; finding the quality of the crèche acceptable and using it; engaging with a group (i.e. informal learning); making friends through Sure Start; engagement in further groups (usually as a result of friends providing mutual support); accessing support from the adult tutor in order to return to adult learning provided by the local FE college and/or to work and/or to volunteering in the local community; planning the next step in learning and/or employment; and having a longer-term plan involving learning and/or employment. Crucially, their journeys included steps that built their social capital, as well as their human capital. Indeed, social capital research suggests that social capital 'generally facilitates economic growth' (Halpern 2005, p.71) and that 'Neighbourhoods with concentrated unemployment perform disproportionately worse than would be expected on the basis of the disadvantage of the individuals within them, and this can be attributed to the lack of connections to the employed and economically advantaged' (p.70). Halpern states that, 'the life chances of disadvantaged individuals can be transformed by the presence in their personal networks of even a single employed individual' (p.313). This suggests that even the first step of the adult learners' journey – engaging with Sure Start – was of importance in improving employability. It also suggests the effectiveness of an approach which encourages and supports adults into education, training and employment, where they can form social networks with aspirational peers and make connections with other adults in employment.

Parents interviewed identified the barriers to learning and/or employment which had affected them prior to the SSLP. These fell into three categories:

- *issues related to learning and employment provision,* such as timing of courses not fitting around childcare responsibilities, unattractive quality of some crèche provision, lack of work-related opportunities and lack of courses offering work experience, and the fact that, for some parents, earnings gained through employment were off-set by tax and reduced benefits (Adam, Brewer and Shephard 2006 provide evidence of the accuracy of the parents' perception that 'For people who get benefits, sometimes it doesn't balance out for them to go back to work if the pay is low')

- *attitudes of self and others*, such as fear of returning to learning or employment because of length of time out of that environment, questioning whether it was possible to study and look after a baby at the same time, unsupportive employers and work colleagues

- *personal circumstances*, such as working full-time making it difficult to access further learning to improve skills, or having full-time caring responsibilities making accessing employment difficult.

The interviewees described the adult tutor as having provided them with one-to-one support in a range of ways tailored to their individual aspirations and addressing their specific barriers: listening to them discussing their hopes, plans and fears; providing information about suitable childcare and relevant learning and employment opportunities; supporting enrolment on courses; offering support with coursework; offering reassurance and encouragement; accompanying them to learning locations; providing practical support around job applications and interview techniques; reflecting back to individuals their strengths and qualities.

These parents identified the supportive aspects of the SSLP which they had particularly valued on their journey as: support from the adult tutor, high quality childcare, confidentiality, supportive friendships, supportive staff, learning opportunities at the centre and information about other local learning and employment opportunities displayed in the centre and, importantly, the lack of pressure ('Sure Start don't push people… They wait for the lead to come from them'). They also valued other supports available locally: the Children's Information Service, the library, adult learning provision with crèche provided, local job opportunities. Not least, they recognised their own motivation to realise their aspirations to improve their own lives and those of their children.

Support from the SSLP throughout each step meant that, when interviewed in 2004, Parent 1 was on course for a job in the childcare sector, Parent 3 had decided to retrain as a teaching assistant, Parent 4 had gained part-time office work, Parent 5 was doing an Open University degree and planned to become a teacher, Parent 6 had a part-time job in retail, Parent 7 was considering training as a classroom assistant and had applied to take a Level 2 English course, Parent 8 was employed part-time in the voluntary sector and was pursuing work-based qualifications. Parent 2, a grandmother, was due to begin a family literacy course so she could better support her grandchildren's education.

Parents' ideas for improving access to local learning and employment opportunities addressed the barriers that remained, despite the SSLP. They welcomed Children's Centres, regarded as providing facilities where every local family could benefit regardless of catchment area. They wished for more local opportunities for Family Learning in local venues, including schools, at times that suited parents; high quality crèche/childcare provision throughout the area; a greater range of work-related and work experience opportunities so that parents could build up the confidence to return to work; and wider availability of one-to-one support, as provided by the SSLP adult tutor. They also argued for removal of the low pay poverty trap.

Evidence of impact

The impact of adopting the 'lifelong learning plus' approach to improving parental employability in Sure Start Chelmsley Wood could be seen in three areas: increased take-up of adult learning by parents, parents becoming employed, and parents becoming involved in improving services and facilities in the local area.

Parents taking up adult learning opportunities

Having begun in late 2000, by 2004 there was evidence of increased take-up of adult learning in Chelmsley Wood from three sources:

- *Activity levels in the SSLP* showed that 681 families (out of 845) had joined as Sure Start members and so were able to access information and support around employment and further learning in the Sure Start building. Of these, 158 individuals had engaged one-to-one with the adult tutor; 67 parents had completed Early Start; 21 had attended Family Literacy and 30 had attended a series of tasters of courses available at the local college.

- *Attendance data supplied by the local FE college* showed that between 1999 (prior to the SSLP) and 2004, the number of families from the Chelmsley Wood area involved in Family Learning increased from 25 to over 300. Although year-on-year figures were not provided, the local FE college reported marked increases in enrolment levels from Chelmsley Wood postcodes (1269 learners on accredited courses in 2003–2004 and 403 on informal courses) describing this as 'really very, very strong...compared to previous years'. College interviewees also reported increased take-up of Level 2 courses by Chelmsley Wood residents. One stated that one-third of the students on one foundation degree course were from Chelmsley Wood.

- *An audit undertaken by the local Learning and Skills Council* (2004) enabled levels of adult participation in learning in the Chelmsley Wood ward to be compared with levels in its adjacent two wards. This showed that there were roughly 7.5 times as many adult learners in the Chelmsley Wood ward compared to the other two.

There was also evidence of individuals progressing from first steps learning to higher levels of learning. SSLP records, although incomplete, showed that at least half of the Sure Start members who received one-to-one support from the adult tutor progressed to various forms of adult learning. Interviews with college staff provided qualitative evidence of individuals' learning progression to supplement the eight case study interviews with parents. Examples included: progression from Family Learning to a foundation degree course; from informal learning to Open College-accredited learning to a university-accredited course; and from Early Start to university degree courses.

Parents becoming employed

Although no figures were obtained, there was evidence from a range of sources that some parents were moving from learning into employment. The eight case studies provided one source. College staff reported that a particularly successful progression route was from Sure Start to foundation degree course in the college and on to employment locally in the childcare sector. They reported knowing of 'many individuals' who had progressed from first steps learning to further education to employment. Local Jobcentre Plus staff regarded the SSLP as a very useful means of supporting parents, particularly lone parents, on their journey to employment, but were unable to provide details of the numbers involved.

Thus it appears that parents were improving their employability by first engaging with Sure Start and, through that, with informal learning. With adult tutor support, they were going on to further learning outside Sure Start, to voluntary work in Sure Start or in the local community, and even to paid employment in chosen areas of work that suited individual aspirations and circumstances.

Parents engaging in community development

The 'lifelong learning plus' approach, grounded in learning conversations and the containment aspect of the Solihull Approach, successfully developed parental agency and empowerment. This was manifested not only in individual progression but also in community-orientated action such as Sure Start parents challenging the quality of crèche provision locally and succeeding in making the provision of high quality affordable childcare a local priority; setting up and running new local playgroups; creating a demand for a wider range of better quality courses accessible to parents; acting as parent representatives on local committees, including those of the college, the local authority and the health trust; and setting up a community action group, Parent Action Community Team (Cullen and Lindsay 2005). Thus, not only were individuals and their families 'strengthened', but also the community.

Conclusion

Whether or not Sure Start Chelmsley Wood Local Programme hit the target 12 per cent reduction in children under four living in workless households – the children may be older before mothers and/or fathers become employed – the benefit of a lifelong learning approach is that these 'skilled-up' adults are more likely to *sustain* employability. Adopting a lifelong learning approach, complemented by active and intermediate labour market approaches, enabled parents to improve their employability across a wide range of individual situations and skill levels – from individuals starting from a position of no formal qualifications and no prior work experience to those who had qualifications and experience but worried about having been out of the job market.

Based on the evidence discussed in this chapter, it seems reasonable, therefore, to suppose that a lifelong learning approach adopted in other settings, such as Children's Centres, will be effective in improving parental employability and thus contribute to breaking the trans-generational cycle of poverty and unemployment. Learning from experience in SSLPs, there are, arguably, three main points that Children's Centres across England would do well to take on board as they support parents moving into education, training and work:

- Children's Centres, Neighbourhood Nurseries and extended schools are all places where Family Learning can be offered, but attention must be paid to accessibility and one-to-one support using an empowering approach such as learning conversations.

- All staff working with families could be trained to recognise and support adult learning needs, for example, through the Step into Learning training and development programme (Sure Start 2007).

- It is important to adopt a strategic approach to adult learning and employability across a local authority so that there is consistency of information and straightforward progression routes; this is enhanced when parent learners are heard at a strategic level.

Acknowledgements

The authors would like to thank Anne Gladstone, adult tutor at Sure Start Chelmsley Wood, and all the Sure Start members who took part in the evaluation, for sharing their views and experiences.

References

Adam, S., Brewer, M. and Shephard, A. (2006) *The Poverty Trade-off: Work Incentives and Income Redistribution in Britain.* Bristol: The Policy Press.

Barnes, J., Leach, P., Sylva, K., Stein, A., Malmberg, L.E. and the Families, Children and Child Care Team (2006) 'Infant care in England: mothers' aspirations, experiences, satisfaction and caregiver relationships.' *Early Child Development and Care 176*, 5, 553–573.

Bradshaw, J. (2006) *A Review of the Comparative Evidence on Child Poverty.* York: Joseph Rowntree Foundation.

Conlon, G. (2005) 'The incidence and outcomes associated with the late attainment of qualifications in the United Kingdom.' *Education Economics 13,* 1, 27–45.

Cullen, M.A. and Lindsay, G. (2005) *Supporting Adults Returning to Learning. Sure Start Chelmsley Wood: Report of the Local Evaluation 2004.* Section 3 (of 4). Coventry: CEDAR, University of Warwick.

Dench, S., Hillage, J. and Coare, P. (2006) *The Impact of Learning on Unemployed, Low-qualified Adults: A Systematic Review.* Department for Work and Pensions Research Report No. 375. Leeds: Corporate Document Services.

Douglas, H. (1999) 'The Solihull Approach: helping health visitors to help families with young children.' *Young Minds Magazine 40,* 19–20.

Douglas, H. and Brennan, A. (2004) 'Containment, reciprocity and behaviour management: preliminary evaluation of a brief early intervention (the Solihull Approach) for families with infants and young children.' *International Journal of Infant Observation 7,* 1, 89–107.

Gallie, D. (2004a) 'Unemployment, marginalization risks and welfare policy.' In D. Gallie (ed.) *Resisting Marginalization: Unemployment Experience and Social Policy in the European Union.* Oxford: Oxford University Press.

Gallie, D. (ed.) (2004b) *Resisting Marginalization: Unemployment Experience and Social Policy in the European Union.* Oxford: Oxford University Press.

Halpern, D. (2005) *Social Capital.* Cambridge: Polity Press.

Harri-Augstein, E.S. and Thomas, L.F. (1991) *Learning Conversations: The S-O-L Way for Personal and Organisational Growth.* London: Routledge and Kegan Paul.

HM Treasury (2000) 'Prudent for a purpose: building opportunity and security for all.' *Spending Review 2000: New Public Spending Plans 2001–2004, Cm 4807.* Norwich: HMSO.

HM Treasury and Department for Education and Skills (2005) *Support for Parents; the Best Start for Children.* Norwich: HMSO.

Jenkins, A. (2006) 'Women, lifelong learning and transitions into employment.' *Work, Employment and Society 20,* 2, 308–328.

Jenkins, A., Vignoles, A., Wolf, A. and Galindo-Rueda, F. (2003) 'The determinants and labour market effects of lifelong learning.' *Applied Economics 35,* 1711–1721.

Labour Party (2005) *Britain Forward Not Back. The Labour Party Manifesto 2005.* London: The Labour Party.

Learning and Skills Council Birmingham and Solihull (2004) 'ACL (Adult and Community Learning) Review Birmingham and Solihull.' Birmingham: Sirius Software Ltd.

Levitas, R. (2004) 'Let's hear it for Humpty: social exclusion, the third way and cultural capital.' *Cultural Trends 13,* 2, 41–56.

McIntosh, S. (2004) 'Skills and unemployment.' In D. Gallie (ed.) *Resisting Marginalization: Unemployment Experience and Social Policy in the European Union.* Oxford: Oxford University Press.

Meadows, P. and Garbers, C. (2004) *Improving the Employability of Parents in Sure Start Local Programmes.* National Evaluation Summary. Nottingham: DfES Publications.

NCH Action for Children on behalf of the Sure Start Partnership (2001) *Sure Start Chelmsley Wood Revised Delivery Plan, September, 1991.* Sutton Coldfield: NCH Action for Children.

Nomaguchi, K.M. and Milkie, M.A. (2006) 'Maternal employment in childhood and adults' retrospective reports of parenting practices.' *Journal of Marriage and Family 68,* 5, 573–594.

Pantazis, C., Gordon, D. and Levitas, R. (eds) (2006) *Poverty and Social Exclusion in Britain. The Millennium Survey.* Bristol: Policy Press.

Ritakallio, V.M. and Bradshaw, J. (2006) 'Family poverty in the European Union.' In J. Bradshaw and A. Hatland (eds) *Social Policy, Employment and Family Change in Comparative Perspective.* Cheltenham: Edward Elgar.

Sure Start Unit and Daycare Trust (2004) *Parents and Work – a Guide for Sure Start Local Programmes.* Nottingham: DfES Publications.

Sure Start (2007) 'Step in to Learning Training.' www.surestart.gov.uk/stepintolearning, accessed on 23 August 2007.

van Wels, F. and Knijn, T. (2006) 'Transitional phase or a new balance? Working and caring by mothers with young children in the Netherlands.' *Journal of Family Issues 27*, 5, 633–651.

Chapter 16

Working with Parents as Colleagues

Matthew Pearson and Ann Martin

This chapter explores perspectives from a local programme which employed parents and helped them to develop the necessary skills to take on roles in both family support and child development. Many joined the programme as volunteers or were the recipients of family support before taking up paid positions within the programme. In this chapter we document the complex identity transitions which local people employed by the programme have made. These local parents, many of whom had accessed the services offered by Sure Start prior to taking up paid employment, were encouraged to become members of a team with a professional identity and focus. The ways in which these parent workers negotiated their sense of difference from the professionals and moved to being accepted in the team are a key focus of this paper. We have also been interested in the changing dynamics that occur when established professionals begin to work collaboratively with colleagues to whom they may previously have offered help in the context of their role in family support. The paper draws on Lave and Wenger's (1991) notions of legitimate peripheral participation to describe the types of learning and identity formation which occurred amongst the individuals within the team.

Theoretical framework: Communities of Practice

Lave and Wenger (1991) have set out an influential way of understanding informal learning and its links with identity and knowledge. They originally used the term 'communities of practitioners' to describe a group of people brought together for a specific purpose and united by a shared set of values, tools and concepts. Wenger later developed the analytic and descriptive scope of this concept into Communities of Practice (Wenger 1999). The argument made by Lave and Wenger is that communities of practice exist everywhere, and it is the undertaking of common activities that enables a group to develop a shared understanding about the practices involved in that particular community. It is not so much that staff members (in this case) learn 'knowledge' or are given training to develop the various attitudes, values or ways of responding to clients that might be desirable in this particular community of practice, but that the development of identities within the place of work is influenced by the degree to which all staff members are able to participate in the conversations about practice.

The Sure Start team displayed the characteristics of a community of practice because they were united behind a relatively well defined set of goals, possessed a set of common tools (assessment frameworks, legal and ethical guidelines, including child protection legislation and professional knowledge), and a common language to describe their interventions. There were of course many differences in approach and style between the health visitors and other professionals and the local workers, but the ways in which these two groups negotiated these differences and were able to work together are precisely the kinds of informal learning through shared exchanges to which Lave and Wenger allude.

A core concept in Community of Practice theory is the movement of new-comers from being legitimate peripheral participants to full members of the group. Initially (and evidence supports this) it is likely that new staff members take a more 'fringe' role whilst they are developing their competence, and are gradually able to become fully participating members at the centre of the group. We demonstrate how this happened later in the chapter.

Context

This section of the chapter examines the key issue of the local nature of the interventions which Sure Start can make and briefly explores how programme thinking has developed at both policy and practice levels to take advantage of this context. We then move on to examine some of the recently published literature about Sure Start and what this might tell us about enabling parents to develop an equal voice as part of a locally based team providing community-led services. The challenge between offering relatively low-paid employment within a Sure Start programme, which may be seen as simply an alternative job with more family-friendly conditions of service, and creating sustainable and meaningful posts which root the aims of initiatives such as Sure Start firmly within communities, is also considered. The extent to which the inclusion of parents as full members of the decision-making workforce can have an impact upon the cultural change of an area also forms part of this discussion.

Gustaffson and Driver (2005) noted that New Labour identified public participation as a key component of delivering services which were more responsive to local communities and contexts and where innovation and creative solutions are expected to flow naturally as a result of the particular per-spectives which the public can bring to bear. They argue that the concepts of hierarchies and markets are being replaced by 'networks', where power and decision-making are wrested away from the 'leaden hand' of central control.

Notions of the 'local' are embedded in the history and genesis of the Sure Start initiative. Glass (1999) writing about the policy history of Sure Start charts the findings of the 'cross-cutting' Comprehensive Spending Review in 2000, which led to the initial investment by New Labour, and notes that one of the recommendations of the review was for an intervention which had a range of characteristics, one of them being: 'locally driven: based on consultation and involvement of parents and local communities' (Glass 1999, p.262). Naomi Eisenstadt, Director of Sure Start, was able to claim three years later that it 'is enormously popular with local parents' (Eisenstadt 2002, p.3). Policy makers were eager to demonstrate that the *locally based* nature of Sure Start Local Programmes (SSLPs) made a difference, particularly in providing services which met the needs of users who may be hard to reach. There is also an emerging body of research and evaluation evidence which finds explanations for the success of various SSLP initiatives in the *local character* of the intervention. For instance, Wigfall (2006), writing about a project called Families in Focus, comments that the setting of the intervention is what made the difference in working with socially excluded families. Jones (2006) also uses an explanation based on the concept of a 'local service' to explain the success of a parenting initiative. There is therefore considerable support for the view that the locally based nature of the SSLP makes a difference, because it is equated with involvement from parents in the area and with their clear support for strategies to improve parenting and the lives of children.

The work in this chapter was conducted at Spa Spiders Sure Start in Askern, which is located near Doncaster in Yorkshire. The area covered by the SSLP was four towns or villages, with Askern being the largest. The area was the site of a large coalmine which was closed in 1991, leading to high rates of unemployment, particularly among men. The area is not ethnically diverse with very few people from ethnic groups other than white. In terms of socioeconomic profile, the area is diverse; there are estates where poverty and deprivation are extremely high, but there are also areas with expensive private houses. The area thus presented a number of challenges to the SSLP, namely the need to tackle poverty and social exclusion caused by high levels of structural unemployment and also the need to create a community resource which was available to all.

An often-cited strength of the Sure Start intervention has been the ways in which SSLPs have been able to meet the needs of local communities because of their sense of being situated within those communities and therefore being more responsive to their needs. This sense of extra responsiveness being invoked here will of course need to be compared to an alternative context or service delivery system, which in this case is that of mainstream services. The contrast between traditional mainstream services and SSLPs can often be quite stark, yet there is more complexity to it than a simple formula which equates SSLPs with local responsiveness and customer focus and dismisses mainstream services as bureaucratic and monolithic and largely ignoring the needs of local people. These stereotypes need to be resisted because SSLPs can sometimes function in much the same way as mainstream services, and there are many examples of mainstream services working creatively in order to embed their services in the communities of local users.

The programme at Askern was developed through the work of a very active and action-oriented group of local parents who collaborated fully on the initial bids and who partnered the SSLP during its early stages and did much to direct the policy and practice during those first years. Representation of local parents on the initial committees for the programme was extremely high, and the setting up of the SSLP was driven by a small but active number of local people. The pattern of local involvement in the programme continued once funding had been secured and around 75 per cent of the paid workers with the programme were taken from the population of local parents. In this case, there-fore, we conclude that the SSLPs grew out of the particular needs of people within the local community. That can set up considerable expectations, not only in terms of the services which parents expect for themselves and their children, but also with respect to development, training and employment opportunities. See Morrow and Malin (2004) for a discussion of how a parents' committee contributed to the management and strategy of an SSLP.

The literature which deals with issues from SSLPs is largely distinct from the National Evaluation of Sure Start (NESS), with the exception of the synthe-sis reports generated by this programme of evaluation. The piecemeal SSLP evaluation literature documents the innovation and learning in which SSLPs have been involved during the life of the initiative. It describes the evidence derived from SSLPs about the kinds of interventions and projects which work with local communities. That part chosen for review here sheds some light on how we might understand the transition which parents make when they become paid employees of Sure Start.

Morrow, Malin and Jennings (2005) evaluated an interprofessional team working in a trailblazer Sure Start and found that considerable tensions surfaced during meetings of the team to discuss the allocation and referral of cases.

> Some staff felt that the nature of their work was leading to them "getting closer" to clients, that "families are offloading more" and that "professional distance is no longer there". Individual staff recognized that they were strug-gling with the tension between traditional practice and different models of working. (Morrow *et al.* 2005, p.97)

This issue of 'distance', the attendant problems of how close the client relation-ship gets, and the tension between different models of working are themes which we observed during this evaluation.

There has also been some exploration of the gendered nature of childcare. Osgood (2005), writing of the government's drive to recruit women into childcare 'careers', commented:

> As such, I would argue that childcare careers are trivialized and positioned as "default" careers that are available to anyone who has some spare time on their hands and unlikely to have the educational and social capital needed to gain "real" employment. (Osgood 2005, p.292)

Some of the Sure Start workers were recruited on to the Askern programme to undertake various positions linked with child development rather than child care, although the broad point made by Osgood may be pertinent to this discussion as it reminds us of the difficulties which local people may have in securing a career for themselves. Most of them lack the transport to get them to larger centres of population where jobs are more abundant. In the SSLP under discussion here, the Sure Start employment option is one of the few available to parents who wish to move beyond unskilled manual jobs and build careers.

Hey and Bradford (2006) have examined the various meanings of motherhood which have emerged through the Sure Start intervention and the ways in which policy discourses are translated into social practices. Their study is rooted both in the context of a local programme but also in the wider issues of identity and knowledge which Sure Start opens up. They conclude that:

> Reconciling your own needs with those of your child, let alone of the community's children, is an ambiguous (and indeed, ambitious) struggle. It avoids that which needs to be seriously tackled in social policy – how do we look after the next generation in a society in which social esteem is solely registered in terms of paid employment? Sure Start offers some resources to think through this conundrum and, as we have seen, some women have clearly thrived in this new partnership. (Hey and Bradford 2006, p.62)

Many of the Askern workers were caught in an even more complex and challenging situation than this, as they had roles both as parents and as paid employees. Their activity within the Sure Start was inextricably bound up in a series of complex issues of identity and practice. During the interviewing a theme which was often brought up was what to do if a parent from the Sure Start stopped a local worker when they were shopping or doing leisure activity in the local community. The local worker was not 'on duty', but as the parents had come to associate them with a source of help and support, the exact etiquette governing these exchanges was unclear. If the worker rejected the advance of the parent and told them to return to the Sure Start to seek help at a more appropriate time then a professional distance would be enacted, but this could also be seen as a source of resentment, and local workers were well aware that a rejection of this kind could cause bad feeling with the very people whom they were hoping to help. Yet to take the other option and engage in family support in the local shop is also fraught with difficulties as the distance between worker and client collapses completely. The workers, who received training in confidentiality and associated legal issues, may be well aware that the 'chat' in the shop may not be as simple as it first appears, and in this example, raised by more than one worker, the issues of identity and professional distance coalesce to create an ethical dilemma which many of the workers were unable to solve.

Methodology

This chapter is founded in a qualitative ethnographic evaluation of the workers at Askern Sure Start who had been recruited from the local community. All Sure Start workers who lived locally were individually interviewed during the course of the research using a semistructured interview format. Questions were grouped thematically and included clusters of questions about how the person came to work for Sure Start, their personal experiences of parenting and of any family support or similar activities, and their aspirations and motivations for developing their career or work profile further. We also interviewed the full-time members of the team who held professional roles, such as the midwives, health visitors and family support workers, in order to set the data from the local workers in context. In addition to the interviewing, we observed the regular meetings of an outreach team where a group of family support workers and health visitors were working together to produce an integrated approach to family support. The observation of meetings enabled us to take 'thick' descriptive accounts of the working practices and day-to-day arrangements which the team developed.

It is customary when recounting observation work to clarify whether the researchers were participant or non-participant, but in this case we occupied a kind of middle ground between these two poles. We participated in meetings in the sense that the team would occasionally ask for our input and we became involved in discussions about team forming and clarification of the values and group identity of the team. But we also spent much of the meetings as passive observers, recording events as they happened and building up a picture of the complex sets of social and cultural practices which shaped these events.

The data were analysed thematically and then a theoretical framework based on the 'community of practice' concept of Lave and Wenger (1991) was applied. This framework describes the kinds of informal learning which happen in groups and how expertise and knowledge is passed from experienced members of the group to new participants. As with all meaningful theoretical frameworks we were able to apply the ideas and concepts both as a lens with which to make sense of a large amount of complex and rich data and as a tool for analysis. This analysis helped to challenge routinised ways of thinking about the attitudes and behaviour of the local parent workers.

Results: 'parent' to 'professional' – states of transition

This section will explore the themes which arose from the study of local parents employed in the SSLP and the issues raised by creating a team comprising both professionals and local parents who are taking their first steps in a skilled job.

Flexibility

A major issue which emerged during the interviewing of the workers centred on employment conditions and the informal arrangements which govern their working lives. The SSLP made great efforts to make conditions child- and family-friendly, with flexible working hours for parents and opportunities to fit working in with school and other commitments. To have done otherwise and enacted a strict regime with little flexibility would have been extremely problematic for the SSLP as in many ways the programme was able to model good practice for other employers in supporting parents in their transition from full-time carers to employees. In addition, it was often the family-orientated aspect of the organisation that encouraged local parents to apply for vacancies. It is questionable whether parents would have been persuaded to apply for jobs if there had been less consideration of their lifestyles. Many parents had previously had to give up paid work as it created practical difficulties when combined with family responsibilities.

> I used to work at C – shift work but it finished at 4.30 and when A started school, I couldn't get anyone to pick her up.

> You've always got to be able to take time off if you've got children haven't you?

> I've had loads of different jobs and most of the time it's been a nightmare trying to fit it all round the kids – this is great here, because we're all in the same boat.

Yet the research revealed this family-friendly approach to be a source of tension between members of the team, some of whom felt that the approach was too flexible and allowed some of the team to escape what we could term 'professional obligations'. These obligations, namely to be in a specific place at a given time in order to meet or work with a client, were part of the core values of the professionally qualified team members, who were often frustrated when they did not see the same commitment and values being enacted by their team members drawn from the local community. There was some feeling that the work was unequally distributed on account of these different levels of commitment. Workers who did not feel it appropriate or possible, given the workload, to adopt a flexible approach to their working patterns commented on this.

> A few of us want school holidays off – we need to have a sort of rota so that leave is shared out fairly.

It's fair enough if some people don't want leave over the summer or whatever, but a lot of us do...and we feel we're always the last to be considered because we do turn up if there's work on whatever our circumstances – that's the difference.

If my daughter is off sick from school, my first thought would be whether her dad could take time off to look after her if I had appointments – you're always thinking you're letting other people down or causing them more work.

However, analysis of the data showed that the perception that some team members played family commitments off against the family-friendly policy of their employer was probably far stronger than the facts warranted. Although some arrangements were made which did allow for flexible working, the true meaning of these arrangements appeared to be symbolic, serving to differentiate the professionalism and 'must do' attitude of the professionals with what was perceived as a more laissez-faire treatment of the local workers.

Autonomy

Autonomy is a high-level skill which builds on a number of others: reflection, observation and the negotiation of personal work in relation to the organisation's strategic goals. It may be applied to time management. For instance, the professional workers appeared to accept what they regarded as an overloaded work schedule as the norm and strove to develop strategies for dealing with this, whereas newer, less experienced members of the staff group did not share this view at all, and did not appear to develop this approach. They had a more functional view of employment, in that the main satisfaction gained was an economic one, and working hours, whilst flexible, did not extend into formal non-working hours.

Most local parents who were workers had held jobs prior to working for Sure Start, but in almost all cases these were unskilled positions, for instance serving in the local bakery or shops. There had often been little opportunity to develop more involved thinking about their work. Clearly the roles created by the SSLP needed levels of autonomy that are needed in other jobs. Our findings showed that autonomy did not appear to arise merely from placing people in a situation where creative and reflective thinking was needed.

Structural differences

There was a clear distinction between those members of the staff group who had professional qualifications (such as health visitors) and the locally recruited parents. All but one of the former group lived outside the catchment area of the Sure Start and frequently recounted the fact that they were glad of this geographic distance between their home environment and their work as this aided in keeping a suitable professional distance between them and their clients. This points to a possible tension between members of the group, one which is structural rather than located within identity or behaviour. The local workers could no more help being local than the health visitors who travelled to a different community to work. The distinction between living and working locally and not living in the community became increasingly important as we analysed the data, and we develop the implications of this distinction in more detail in the section which follows. In addition to location, other factors which have emerged as significant are the ways in which the link between employment and identity are seen, and the interpretation of the values of the 'professional' worker, in terms of the internal expectations often associated with this role.

Confidentiality

The nature of their employment meant that local workers were often in possession of sensitive information about families in the area and this creates a set of ethical dilemmas quite different from those of the professionals who worked but did not live in the area. One simple challenge was to create a necessary professional identity which meant that information was not shared inappropriately or used to gossip about certain families. But another challenge was when a local worker, through their position in the community, knew even more about a particular family and its issues than the professionals did. The issue then became what to do with this knowledge. Sharing it with the group would enhance decision-making processes and potentially it could lead to a crucial intervention with a family, but because the information was gained by the worker outside of the professional context, its status was unclear. Local workers were wrestling with these thorny problems on a regular basis and it was clear that, although the training they received was excellent and they were quick to praise it, there were many situations in which formal training simply could not provide solutions or possible courses of action.

Boundaries

There was evidence too of the professional workers experiencing dilemmas associated with the inclusion of local parents as members of the Family Support Team. Not infrequently, a family, who were friends of one or more of the parent employees, presented with a problem, occasionally of a serious nature. Because there was an awareness that living in the local community could present difficulties, some discussions about particular families were kept within a smaller subgroup of the team to protect colleague parents from experiencing any conflict of interest. This was particularly demonstrated when a local worker's sister-in-law was involved in a potential child protection issue.

> Well I wouldn't like a member of my family to be talked about in front of me. I know it's all our job, but it might make things difficult between all of us.

> She [a local parent colleague] sees that family all the time – they go drinking together – you can't always be clear what you've said when you've had a few…best not to put her in a difficult position I think.

While this strategy was clearly adopted with the intention of relieving potential stress on the part of fellow members of the team, it did in fact lead to extra workload and responsibility for those workers who were party to the information. In addition, the perception of the need to filter information in this way appeared to undermine the idea of team working, and the identity of a cohesive, supportive team environment.

Family support work can be extremely stressful and emotionally intensive and the need to share details with colleagues is one way of relieving this stress. This route was often thought to be unavailable to some of the professionally trained workers, and the effects were seen as both adding to the pressure of the work, and creating divisions within the team, further separating the established workers from the newer staff members drawn from the local area.

In addition to the possible divisions created by an awareness of the extensive personal neighbourhood links which local parent colleagues had, some of the newer members of staff had themselves received family support at an earlier time, occasionally provided by some of their new colleagues. Although professional values were clearly in evidence (setting boundaries, renegotiating patterns of communication to confirm changed relationships) evidence remained of the challenges that such previous connections sometimes brought to individuals and the team as a whole.

> We often talk about…you know laugh about some families…you just have to sometimes, and then I see her looking and I think she wonders if we ever talked about her like that.

> I feel I have to be strictly professional at all times – I never let myself out of role – I always behave as though I am in front of families.

> I think it creates a sort of stilted tension sometimes. You can never really relax – it's quite hard – we all get on but we've got our own one or two people we let go with.

> I think I'm telling her about this family and it's similar to her situation then [name] makes me feel uncomfortable.

Communities of Practice in action

As the analysis of the data proceeded, we identified a strong theme centred around the difference between the professional and the personal as identity markers, and in the section which follows we develop this notion in relation to Lave and Wenger's Community of Practice (Lave and Wenger 1991).

During the interviews and observations there was evidence that many of the local workers were making this transition from the fringe to full participation in the staff group and learning effectively from the practices of the group and the more experienced members of the team. Many of the workers were able to share their experiences of discussing families as 'cases' where the level and nature of intervention was decided during meetings and where a professional framework of judgements was applied in order to identify the best ways of intervening.

> I used to dread those meetings…thought I might be asked something I didn't know, but now I can see that I might know something about a family or something that the others won't know.

> I think I've learned a lot about their roles [Health Visitors]…not what I thought and I don't feel…no I do feel more on a footing with them. I definitely think we're a whole team working together.

> I'm close to the views of lots of the families we deal with. I'm one of them, I know what a lot of the issues are from first hand experience. I think that has been useful in what I can bring to my job and I think they can see that.

But we also found evidence that the movement from peripheral to central participation could be problematic as the dynamics of the team sometimes worked against full participation. The reasons for this appear to be rooted in the differing identities of the health visitors and the local workers and in a difference in perspective between the two groups. This difference grew out of the conceptual boundaries between the professionals and workers and privileged the professional viewpoint on the correct way of doing family support.

The existence of accepted power structures was clearly evident in some of the formal meetings, and also in the largely unchallenged acceptance of what actually constituted family support – in this case a model of one-to-one intervention with a worker taking on a family as a 'case', diagnosing the steps needed to improve family life, and then helping the family achieve this goal. The model for interaction with families was often influenced by the interventionist perspective and the one-to-one support that this approach might engender. Other forms of family support, such as group work, or accompaniment/befriending, exemplified by supported attendance at specific parenting sessions, appeared to hold less status. Local parent team members felt most confident with the latter approach and it was occasionally difficult to achieve a shared view of the team's functions. The tension between enabling parents to seek help or advice and proactively giving such help was also apparent. Despite the evidence found of a Community of Practice, the core view of family support remains largely unaddressed.

Once again, we can point to a structural issue here. The simple fact that many of the workers had been the recipients of family support themselves and had then crossed over into the role of paid workers meant they found it harder to use a discourse of professional objectivity, and in many cases, because the families under discussion were known personally by the local workers, they found themselves less able to offer judgements on the best course of action because of this lack of professional distance.

While (1998) discusses problems with the issue of empowerment in relation to community nursing and health visiting and reflects on the fact that people cannot be empowered by a third party; they have to take the steps towards self-determination themselves. In some ways this tension was being played out within the local workers in the SSLP. They were being placed in a position where they could empower themselves by developing a career in family support but this was not a straightforward task, as illustrated by the issues revealed by our analysis: flexibility, autonomy, structural considerations, confidentiality and boundaries.

The existence of family-friendly policies in order to recognise the often conflicting roles of parent and worker is, we argue, necessary to encourage local parents to feel they could apply for such work in the first place. In addition, flexible ways of working which can help parents absorb some of the pressures of their dual responsibilities are needed if these members of the community are to be encouraged into family support roles. In the wider context of encouraging the educational and occupational development of local parents, care needs to be taken to ensure that realistic expectations of the role of employee are engendered by the notion of obligation and responsibility to the workplace and colleagues. Failure to do this may lead to dissatisfaction amongst the wider staff group as we have reported, in that a dual approach to work roles and expectations is allowed to develop which favours one group over another. In addition, the understandable desire to use incentives of flexibility to encourage parents to take on work roles which may previously have not been thought of as an option may conversely lead to the same parents experiencing arrested occupational development, by virtue of the fact that their work conditions are far more favourable than could reasonably be expected elsewhere.

> This is my dream job, I'd never want to leave it. It's so handy, on the doorstep, I can take B to school and pick her up...can take M with me a lot of the time.

> When I saw there were jobs coming up I was really excited. It's great to have work like this just down the road, nice atmosphere to work in and everything, we're nearly all local, and we all go out a lot and have a laugh. I can't see me moving on.

> I've told L to come along and volunteer at [SSLP]...she'd love a job here too, she's always saying I've landed on my feet here.

Family-friendly working conditions may be a disincentive to moving. While this may not be a problem for individual parents who have achieved the level of occupational development they desire, it may limit the opportunities open to other local parents, in that once the initial jobs for local parents are filled there is very little movement in later years. Communities of Practice develop most dynamically when new members are incorporated into them, and a largely static membership may impede the evolution of practice.

Conclusion

Our research with the local workers at Askern Sure Start underlined some key developmental issues from which any similar teams or ventures may learn. The first and most important conclusion we reached is that the identity of both individuals and a team is a crucial element of success. Whilst suggesting that a group can be brought together and immediately begin working together productively is naive when described, all too often this assumption is made implicitly. The result is the formation of teams with little attention paid to the ways in which the identity of individuals will be both mediated through their interaction with the group and in many cases radically altered as a result of their immersion in a Community of Practice.

We have conceptualised professionalism in this chapter as a state of relative detachment from clients, although this distance is frequently challenged. Moving to a state of professional engagement is about far more than acquiring a set of discrete skills and applying them in practice. It is rather about significant shifts in self-identity which take place as the result of encounters with new social practices, language and situations. It may be too much to expect local parents to make the transition to professionalism without an explicit focus on identity issues as part of their training, but also with the realisation that much of the learning they will undertake will be implicit and tacit, hidden in a complex web of social relations.

There may sometimes be a need to help to move local workers out of what we term their 'comfort zones'. We observed that some parents found a role in the programme undertaking tasks they were comfortable with, but were reluctant to take on further responsibilities. In Lave and Wenger's terms they were resisting the move to central participation and holding on to their status as peripheral participants.

The ethos of community-driven initiatives is well evidenced as the most effective way of encouraging cultural change and evolution. Placing parents at the centre of initiatives has engaged many people. The changing perception of parents about living in Askern and the surrounding district is partly due to their awareness that their views can influence the services offered, but is also related to the fact that they can directly affect the provision and delivery of local services by being central to the process of decision-making and service delivery. The traditional knowledge hierarchy (the top-down approach) is likely to be less relevant in the development of peer-led services where appropriate knowledge may be held by different members of a group at any one time, and therefore a range of roles needs to played by all: followers, team players, leaders and subject experts.

Implications for Children's Centres

- Hierarchical structures that favour professional status need to adapt to involve parents fully.

- Management should foster the informal learning that arises spontaneously from participating in a community of practice.

- Children's Centres should be aware of the complex interface between the needs of a particular community and the aims, objectives and targets of a professionally led service.

Acknowledgements

We would like to thank the staff of Spa Spiders Sure Start in Askern for taking part in the evaluation activity which led to this chapter and in particular the programme manager, Pam Ley, whose support has been very important.

References

Eisenstadt, N. (2002) 'Sure Start key principles and ethos.' Child Care, Health and Development 28, 1, 3–4.

Glass, N. (1999) 'Sure Start: the development of an early intervention programme for young children in the United Kingdom.' Children and Society 13, 57–264.

Gustaffson, U. and Driver, S. (2005) 'Parents, power and public participation: Sure Start, an experiment in New Labour governance.' Social Policy and Administration 39, 5, 528–543.

Hey, V. and Bradford, S. (2006) 'Re-engineering motherhood? Sure Start in the community.' Contemporary Issues in Early Childhood 7, 1, 54–67.

Jones, L. (2006) 'Developing everyone's learning and thinking abilities: a parenting programme – the Southern area experience 10 years on!' Child Care in Practice 1, 2, 141–155.

Lave, J. and Wenger, E. (1991) Situated Learning. Legitimate Peripheral Participation. Cambridge: Cambridge University Press.

Morrow, G. and Malin, N. (2004) 'Parents and professionals working together: turning the rhetoric into reality.' Early Years 24, 2, 163–177.

Morrow, G., Malin, N. and Jennings, T. (2005) 'Interprofessional teamworking for child and family referral in a Sure Start setting.' Journal of Interprofessional Care 19, 2, 93–101.

Osgood, J. (2005) 'Who Cares? The classed nature of childcare.' Gender and Education 17, 3, 289–303.

Wenger, E. (1999) Communities of Practice. Learning, Meaning and Identity. Cambridge: Cambridge University Press.

While, A. (1998) 'Is Sure Start good for health visiting?' British Journal of Community Nursing 3, 10, 519.

Wigfall, V. (2006) 'Bringing back community: family support from the bottom up.' Children and Society 20, 17–29.

Part 4

Supporting Families

Chapter 17

Introduction to Supporting Families

Mark Avis

In identifying the background to the support for families offered within Sure Start programmes, we should recognise two interrelated issues that have helped to shape services: a shift towards a social investment model of welfare and a shift away from the view that childcare is the sole responsibility of the family. The social investment model promotes the idea that social welfare should be accomplished through the development of individual and community resources rather than through the direct provision of economic maintenance (Giddens 1998). A central aspect of Sure Start initiatives has been to address the consequences of children growing up in areas with a record of patchy childcare and poorly integrated family support services, and where many of the families who are in need of support may distrust statutory services and government agencies. Therefore, Sure Start Local Programmes were expected to implement ways of providing services that would reach out to vulnerable families and support their parenting, as well as enhancing the availability and quality of local child care and family support and removing some of the embedded barriers to accessing services (Tunstill *et al.* 2005).

Part 4 of this book provides some illustrations of the way in which Sure Start Local Programmes have attempted to deliver improved family support. At the heart of each Sure Start Local Programme was a core offer of family support services that would be provided. These core services included home visits, providing information and support on children's emotional and social development, support for the development of parenting skills, referral to specialist services, increasing the involvement of fathers, and parenting support for families identified as 'hard-to-reach'. As we have observed elsewhere in this book, Sure Start Local Programmes had no national blueprint to follow. Each Sure Start Local Programme tried to develop its own model of service to address a range of targets that included: engagement with 'harder to reach' families, use of residential care, identification and support of vulnerable families, and registrations on the child protection register. In most cases, Local Programmes have worked to emphasise the supportive, befriending and pre-ventative aspects of family support that made their services different from, but integrated with, existing statutory services. Effective collaboration between health and social care agencies based on information sharing and mutual understanding is regarded as essential in providing services to families with multiple disadvantages and preventing children becoming at risk.

However, some difficulty remains in stating the nature and defining characteristics of family support. Chapter 18 by Thurston focuses on the provision of preventative support to families and provides a picture of how professionals attempted to deliver a service that made family support responsive to parents' needs and facilitative of parental change. Crosbie and Avis in Chapter 19 draw attention to another aspect of preventative family support through the provision of a respite scheme in association with local nurseries. Barton, Jesson and Horton in Chapter 22 review some of the core values of family support, and highlight the difficulties of evaluating family support services when there is a lack of consensus regarding these core values. They draw attention to the need to have a clear theoretical framework for the provision of family support services, and argue that it will remain difficult to evaluate the effectiveness of family services provided by Children's Centres until we have more clarity about what services are trying to achieve. As Thurston illustrates, evaluation can demonstrate process outputs in terms of improved relationships between professionals and families, and increased readiness and confidence to change behaviours, but it remains an elusive goal to show how family support services have led to a range of particular evaluation outcomes. Barton, Jesson and Horton point out that the complexity of the problems faced by families, the fairly rapid movement of families in and out of Sure Start areas, and changes in Sure Start services as they evolve in response to local family demands, mean that it may take many more years to get to really understand what makes a difference in family support services.

It is noticeable that a key feature of many Sure Start Local Programmes is the use of 'outreach' services. The concept is interesting because it captures the way in which Sure Start embodies a break with the 'equity of access' model that informs how many existing services are provided. The idea of reaching out to particular families and people in need of support indicates a shift from the values of universal, equitable and impartial professional support that are thought to underpin statutory services. The use of outreach in Sure Start Local Programmes places an emphasis on a more particular, more personal, way of reaching out and interacting with people in need of support. However, the concept of outreach is often associated with the idea of 'hard-to-reach' groups. The label of 'hard-to-reach' has been subject to some criticism because it seems to place the responsibility for any failure to become involved with services with the parents themselves. One group of parents who have suffered the consequences of being labelled 'hard-to-reach' has been fathers. McKenna in Chapter 21 explores the way that Sure Start Programmes have addressed the involvement of fathers. She reinforces the idea that inclusion of fathers is essential in meeting Sure Start goals and provides illustrations of how Sure Start has helped some fathers rethink their role in the family and talk about fatherhood in new ways, but she also challenges some of the ways in which fathers' participation has been addressed in Sure Start programmes.

A further aspect of the idea of outreach has been the recognition that services must be relevant, attractive and non-judgemental. However, an aspect of outreach that requires further attention is the way it is requiring health and social care professionals to incorporate the idea of 'befriending' into their practice. Thurston suggests that this more informal and less judgemental way of delivering family support has resulted in a less 'directive' approach to support. Featherstone, Manby and Nicholls explore this emergent theme further in Chapter 20 and examine the consequences of these new types of relationships between professionals and service users, and how the tensions around being a friend, being friendly, and managing dependence are negotiated.

It would seem that there remains scope for much further evaluation of the nature of family support in the context of children's centres. As demonstrated in the evaluations described in these chapters, considerable learning amongst professionals associated with Sure Start Local Programmes has occurred in the process of shifting the perceptions of family support services, through the emphasis on outreach, social investment, and in developing models of professional–client relationships that can accommodate the concept of befriending. This learning needs to be sustained by children's centres if they are to fulfil their purpose, and the evaluation studies that inform how these processes have been accomplished will also need to be maintained. However, there remains a major task for future evaluation to provide the evidence that helps to clarify and describe the nature of family support and suggest how its impact on families can be assessed.

References

Giddens, A. (1998) *The Third Way: The Renewal of Social Democracy.* Cambridge: Polity Press.

Tunstill, J., Allnock, D., Akhurst, S., Garbers, C. and the Ness Research Team (2005) 'Sure Start Local Programmes: implications of case study data from the National Evaluation of Sure Start.' *Children and Society 19*, 2, 158–172.

Chapter 18

Understanding Family Support

Miranda Thurston

Supporting families in deprived areas has been a primary concern of Sure Start Local Programmes. Family support and parental outreach, alongside early education integrated with childcare, and child and family health services together constitute the 'core offer' of Sure Start Children's Centres (Sure Start 2005) — that is to say, all Sure Start funded Children's Centres must offer these services. Yet there is considerable debate about what constitutes family support and how it should be delivered, particularly within the context of developing early preventative models of provision (King's Fund 2004).

This chapter explores the concept of family support by considering some of the findings from the local evaluation of family support provision in one Sure Start Local Programme (Pearson and Thurston 2006). The aim of the chapter is to consider how the local programme operationalised the concept of family support by seeking to identify the characteristic features of its provision. The chapter also considers the impact of this model of family support by exploring the ways in which being supported led to changes in families' circumstances. The chapter sheds light on the ways in which a Sure Start Local Programme has responded to the policy imperative of creating early preventative services, within the context of the expressed needs of the local population, and considers the implications of the findings for the provision of family support within Sure Start Children's Centres.

Methodology

An exploratory case study approach was used in order to understand how family support was provided by the Sure Start Local Programme and with what kinds of consequences. This approach used a number of qualitative methods to generate rich descriptions of service processes and user experiences in order to build up a picture of how professionals delivered family support, how this was experienced by families, and with what kinds of consequences (Pearson and Thurston 2006). The following fieldwork was carried out:

1. in-depth interviews with 12 Sure Start staff (from a team of 19) who had a primary role in providing family support

2. in-depth interviews with 20 parents who had experienced family support

3. observation of five core services, which were identified as making a major contribution to family support (the Pop In, the Drop In, the Parenting Programme, adult education, and pre-birth experience)

4. observation of home visits and one-to-one sessions with five different Sure Start workers (the play development worker, the two Sure Start midwives, two of the three Sure Start family support workers).

The in-depth interviews with Sure Start staff and parents were transcribed verbatim and analysed thematically. The observations were used to build up descriptions of the different forms of service delivery and the different types of interactions that took place. This allowed the interview data to be interpreted in context.

Ethical approval was granted by South Cheshire Local Research Ethics Committee in December 2003.

Findings

The qualitative material from all the fieldwork was used to reveal:

1. the characteristics of the model underpinning family support provision in terms of what services were provided and what support activities were carried out, by whom and in what ways

2. the nature of the family support relationship between parents and Sure Start staff

3. the ways in which family support led to changes in family circumstances and functioning.

The Sure Start Local Programme's model of family support

It was possible to understand the model of family support in terms of the organisation of provision that defined the ways in which parents could access support, and the kinds of services and support that were available. Family support was provided through five core services: two of these services – the Pop In and the Drop In – operated on an informal basis; the other three – the Parenting Programme, adult education, and pre-birth experience – operated on a more structured basis. Home visiting was also available, either to deliver these core services in the home or to provide individualised one-to-one support around specific issues. Ad hoc informal advice and support was provided in both structured settings and the home.

Families came to access support by a process of referral, referrals being discussed at the weekly allocations meeting attended by all staff, where decisions were made about which member of staff would support the family. It was evident that these decisions were made on the basis of a combination of factors relating to: individuals' knowledge of the family, the nature of the particular issue around which support was needed, workloads of staff, and the skills of individual team members. Alongside this formal process ran an informal one that had emerged in an effort to respond quickly to self-referrals (often from families who had not had any previous contact with the local programme) and referrals from within the Sure Start team. Once allocated, the member of staff would make contact with the family to arrange a visit to explore how best the family could be supported. This could be through any combination of the above services and support activities, and for any duration. Staff reported that support was there for as long as a family needed it.

At the time of the fieldwork, family support was provided by a multidisciplinary team of 19. It was evident from the interviews that all Sure Start workers were seen as having a role in providing family support. However, those staff with an involvement in the five core services were specifically identified as having a central role in supporting families: three family support workers, one health visitor, two midwives, one play development worker, one adult learning coordinator, two nursery nurses and the deputy programme manager (who was also a community development worker). From this description it is evident that family support did not operate as one distinct service within the programme (Pearson and Thurston 2006). Rather, the model developed was one in which the primary aim of all work and interaction with families was to support them in ways that met their expressed needs, and with the ultimate aim of benefiting the child. For example, one member of staff said: 'Everyone, in a sense, delivers family support because we all provide advice and support to enable parents to bring up their children...everyone is part of that picture'.

Providing family support through a multidisciplinary team was perceived by staff as a positive aspect of Sure Start provision but one which also had its challenges. On the positive side, the view was expressed by staff that the team could respond promptly to the diverse and often complex needs of parents, often without the necessity of involving other agencies. This meant that the role of supporting families in complex situations could be shared across the team. Furthermore, working in this way meant that staff had a better understanding of the range of factors affecting families and were better able to provide a holistic, family-centred response. However, the view was expressed that it had taken time to adjust to working in an integrated team within a community setting, particularly in terms of embracing new, more generic and low-level ways of working as part of a specialist role (Pearson and Thurston 2006). In part, this was about how the different professional disciplines within the team were utilised to provide coherent and effective support. Some staff thought that all professionals in the team could address any family support issue unless it was 'really complicated'; others talked about the need to utilise specialist skills appropriately so that things 'didn't get missed'. For example, one professional stated:

> For me family support has been the hardest service to understand…you could still work very independently here if we were not careful…in the early days I used to think family support was the answer to everything and actually realised that a lot of the stuff that I do within midwifery is family support.

The issue of professional identity and boundaries was thought to be particularly unclear in relation to the work of the family support workers and nursery nurses. Family support workers were seen by some team members to have the time to provide cross-cutting support to families because they did not have a specialist role (like a midwife, for example). Family support workers themselves saw their role focusing on work with families who were in contact with social services and in providing specialist welfare advice, but this was not a universal team view. Some team members viewed nursery nurses as key to family support provision, as the following quotation illustrates:

> The nursery nurses are almost crucial to the whole process here because what they do is they actually belong to nearly everything…they are crucial to family support because they help so many of us with our work… I would call them family support workers.

Family support was provided in relation to a range of issues and in a variety of ways. Thus, parents and staff talked about family support in terms of:

1. advice and guidance, for example in respect of claiming benefits to which they were entitled, improving safety in the home, breastfeeding, and speech and language advice

2. emotional support, for example, listening to parents' problems, talking through personal issues of concern, helping them through crises and transitions

3. befriending, particularly in cases where individuals were very isolated and had no-one on whom they could call

4. advocacy, in situations where contact with other agencies or organisations was required and the parent's case was put forward for him/her

5. practical support, in terms of managing day-to-day tasks and routines, providing transport to attend appointments, help with form-filling and collecting prescriptions

6. developing parenting skills, in terms of helping parents develop their relationship with their child through assisting with aspects of behaviour, including sleeping, bed-wetting and potty-training

7. direct work with children, particularly in respect of play and behaviour

8. working with complex families, with multiple issues and often involving sustained support from several agencies that required coordination

9. supporting parents with mental health problems who had been unable to access support from other agencies

10. facilitating access to statutory services, such as social services, in respect of child protection issues.

Such multifaceted provision illustrates that family support was provided along a continuum, from fairly low-level support at one end of the spectrum through to quite high-level and intense support at the other (Pearson and Thurston 2006).

The nature of the relationship between families and Sure Start staff

In talking about family support, both parents and professionals made comparisons with how services had been delivered by other organisations of which they had some experience. Professionals tended to describe their role within the Sure Start team in terms of developing positive relationships with parents and facilitating family life (Pearson and Thurston 2006). For professionals, carrying out family support in a non-threatening, non-stigmatising way that avoided victim-blaming was important if families were to be successfully engaged. For example, one professional said: 'People see us...as somebody they can chat to confidentially [who] is not going to make judgements'.

A further aspect of developing non-stigmatising, non-threatening family support related to the informal and low-key nature of the interactions between parents and staff even within the context of more structured settings. It was evident that this way of working generated opportunities for parents to raise their concerns with staff, and for staff to respond through the everyday processes of interaction (Pearson and Thurston 2006). There was also evidence to suggest that staff did not present themselves as the experts with all the answers. For example, parents talked about Sure Start staff in terms of not 'lecturing' or 'dictating' to them, but, rather, offering suggestions and being prepared to try other approaches if things failed. Professionals thought that this approach had been particularly successful in responding to parenting issues, as one commented:

> I definitely think families appreciate the fact that somebody will listen and be able to keep going back rather than just to say, "Do this, do that!" and then leave them to it. To have somebody support them and say, "Right! This didn't work, so how about trying it this way?" can be really valuable.

Developing relationships with parents was seen by staff in terms of making an investment of time, time which was often thought not to be available to other professionals. Staff talked about not leaving parents 'high and dry' and of acting in ways which made it evident to parents that they could be relied upon, trusted and would not be blamed for the things that happened to them. It was evident that this affective aspect of interaction was communicated to parents; one parent commented that: 'they understand that things happen and they don't hold it against you'. Investing time in the family support relationship had enabled some parents to continue receiving support from the Sure Start Local Programme when other agencies had withdrawn. For example, one parent commented: 'Sure Start are the only people who haven't deserted me…the social workers did and I don't see much of my health visitor'.

Parents' experiences of interacting with Sure Start staff were described in ways which suggested that staff were able to establish a relationship based on the notion of needs-led support rather than professionally led intervention. For example, they talked about the way in which staff would return their calls, address issues *they* raised and visit at home when *they* wanted them to. The one issue that was described by parents as not being approached helpfully was breastfeeding, which may reflect the sensitivity of the issue for mothers as well as how it is broached by staff. However, overwhelmingly, parents articulated the view that staff were friendly, kind, straightforward, honest, and nice to them, and suggested that their interaction with other professionals was not always characterised by such a degree of warmth. For example, one parent said: 'She talks nice to us and that…not many people talk nice to me'.

Changing family circumstances

Family support was often the first contact with the local programme for families and there was evidence to suggest that relationships between Sure Start staff and parents were such that when support was offered, it was taken up in a sustained way. This meant that establishing a relationship with parents that was based on a degree of mutual understanding created the conditions within which it was possible to bring about change in families' circumstances. Given the relative ease and frequency with which families could access staff, early intervention to address small but important issues became possible and decreased the likelihood of crises engulfing families (Pearson and Thurston 2006). Rather than focusing on parenting skills directly, staff often worked with parents to build a family's capacity to function at times of difficulty through the development of their personal resources, and by addressing practical concerns.

Parents talked positively about the support provided, which they perceived as contributing to a range of constructive outcomes for themselves and their children. When parents and professionals talked about the benefits of engaging

with family support they talked about this in respect of small chan
the potential to make large differences to family circumstances (P
Thurston 2006). For example, advice and guidance from the Sure
was seen as potentially helpful in improving family life. One parent talked
about this in respect of establishing a child's sleeping patterns and another
about improving a child's behaviour, as the following quotation illustrates:

> He wouldn't go in his pushchair. They helped me to try things. They said it is
> OK for him to walk providing he holds my hand but if he didn't it was
> straight in the pushchair, without a warning and then you have to explain why
> you have put him there…it worked and we don't have that hassle now.

Family support could be seen as a process for facilitating change at the level of
the individual. Increasing self-esteem and confidence and reducing anxiety
were frequently alluded to by parents. How parents felt about themselves as
parents was expressed as being important in terms of preventing them from
feeling overwhelmed and unable to cope. Sometimes quite a high level of
support was provided before parents were able to act independently. For
example, one parent said:

> [Member of staff] used to do a lot of home visits and she helped me tremen-
> dously because I suffered a lot with depression and anxiety…we worked well
> together as a team…once she had come here for a while she would meet me
> and come with me to the groups and then now I'm at the stage when I can go
> by myself… I am so much more confident…two years on I don't have the
> home visits any more.

Improvements in confidence and self-esteem were sometimes related to
learning new skills and this, in turn, had the potential to influence family life
positively. For example, one mother talked about the way she had worked on
her parenting skills and routines with a member of Sure Start staff with the following consequences:

> We work on time-outs and things like that…we had a week of hell when
> time-outs first started, he would refuse to go on the bottom step. Now he just
> goes…it is heaven. It is perseverance… I don't think I would have bothered
> with anything like that if it hadn't been for Sure Start helping me… I have
> definitely got more coping skills… I don't find myself as strung out and
> stressed with things any more… I am a lot happier and so is my little boy.

The interdependence between children's behaviour, parental resources to carry
out their parenting role and family dynamics was often described by parents
and staff and it was evident that taking a family-centred approach to issues
could have far-reaching consequences for all family members and their wider
social relationships. For example, one professional said:

> The family who bed-share and whose little girl wet the bed every night…just
> by sorting out that one small thing there have been dramatic changes. She

doesn't have to change her sheets in the middle of the night...so she is getting more sleep. So she feels better in the morning which gave her the confidence to go out. So she takes her daughter to nursery now and mixes with other mums...just that has made a massive difference to their lives.

Discussion

The findings presented above suggest that the Sure Start Local Programme has implemented a model of support that can be described as complex, multifaceted and responsive to families' diverse needs. Given the complexity of families' lives, it is important to understand family support not as a 'one off' event but as a process in which parents' engagement is voluntarily secured (Artaraz and Thurston 2006). The findings from this study would suggest that the nature of the relationship developed between staff and families is of primary importance. In this study, families valued their relationships with professionals, a finding that has been described elsewhere (Artaraz and Thurston 2006; Weinberger 2003). Thus, staff are the vehicles through which engagement is facilitated.

If parents are viewed as experts about their own situation, they are more likely to be listened to – a prerequisite for providing a needs-led response. Listening is also the departure point for providing a flexible and effective response; since families' needs are likely to vary, so too should the support which is offered to them (Pearson and Thurston 2006). This point perhaps cannot be emphasised too strongly and has resonance for the provision of all community-based services aimed at early intervention. Providing informal opportunities for parents to express their needs has the potential to redistribute power in their favour, towards more collaborative styles of support (Mackean, Thurston and Scott 2005; Statham and Holtermann 2004), as it reduces the necessity for professional identification of problems associated with the surveillance of families, and generates the basis for a more trusting relationship. Thus, if professionals base their practice on an approach that is underpinned by the empathic understanding of families and their circumstances, it is likely that the victim-blaming mentality that is so corrosive of parent–professional relationships is avoided. It is also possible that family support can then be presented as a generic, non-issue-based service. This also allows for the possibility of outcomes being achieved through an indirect, rather than a direct, pathway; thus, the needs of the child are seen within the context of the needs of the family (Mackean *et al.* 2005).

This analysis puts the role of staff in engaging and supporting families centre stage. The provision of a multidisciplinary team was beneficial to families because it meant that the local programme had the capacity and capability to respond to the diverse issues that they presented. Despite the perceived value of this approach amongst staff and service users, there were some tensions amongst staff who were perhaps more used to working within much tighter professional boundaries (Pearson and Thurston 2006). These related to the dynamics within the multidisciplinary team as they sought to operationalise this model of family support. The development of integrated professional practice in the provision of family support raises questions about the appropriate balance between role development of all staff and the creation of specialist family support workers, an issue which has resonance for family support work and multidisciplinary working within Children's Centres in the future.

In respect of outcomes, staff are also the vehicles through which outcomes can be mediated. The findings from this research suggest that, when families engaged with family support, there were three ways in which their circumstances could be improved. First, attending to the practical realities of everyday family life can provide some respite from the stress of bringing up children in circumstances of material disadvantage. Moreover, this is an example of the way in which the local programme responded to families' expressed needs; families' priorities were found to revolve around practicalities, not parenting issues, consistent with recent research (Edwards *et al.* quoted in ESRC 2006). Second, the quality of family dynamics can be shifted in a positive direction by advice about, and support for, relatively small issues associated with the behaviour of children (Pearson and Thurston 2006). Finally, resources within the family were found to increase through directly supporting parents in their own personal development – as individuals and as parents – leading to improvements in self-esteem and confidence. If family support is multifaceted, there is a greater likelihood of change being mediated through the cumulative impact of small positive changes.

Implications for Children's Centres

Children's Centres will need to consider how best to integrate such a model into their provision in a way which preserves the emphasis on early, preventative support and presents provision as non-judgemental and non-stigmatising. Given the centrality of professional practice in this type of provision, consideration will need to be given to the following:

1. how to develop a multidisciplinary team that has an adequate mix of specialist and generic expertise, appropriately blended within individual roles

2. how to develop staff to work in a family-centred way, given that many staff working in Children's Centres will not have had the Sure Start experience.

Acknowledgement

I would like to acknowledge the work of Charlotte Pearson as well as all the parents and staff who contributed to the local evaluation. The local evaluation was funded by Sure Start Blacon.

References

Artaraz, K. and Thurston, M. (2006) *A Review of Family Support Provision in Three Sure Start Local Programmes in Halton*. Chester: University of Chester, Centre for Public Health Research.

ESRC Society Today (2006) *Parents Want Concrete Support not Parenting Lessons.* www.esrcsocietytoday.ac.uk/ESRCInfoCentre/PO/releases/2006/september/parents.aspx, accessed on 8 September 2006.

King's Fund (2004) *Finding Out What Works*. London: King's Fund.

Mackean, G.L., Thurston, W.E. and Scott, C.M. (2005) 'Bridging the divide between families and health professionals' perspectives on family-centred care.' *Health Expectations 8*, 74–85.

Pearson, C. and Thurston, M. (2006) *Understanding the Concept of Family Support Provided by Integrated Multi-disciplinary Teams*. Chester: University of Chester, Centre for Public Health Research.

Statham, J. and Holtermann, S. (2004) 'Families on the brink: the effectiveness of family support services.' *Child and Family Social Work 9*, 155–166.

Sure Start (2005) *A Sure Start Children's Centre for Every Community. Phase 2 Planning Guidance (2006–2008)*. www.surestart.gov.uk/_doc/P0000457.doc, accessed on 6 November 2007.

Weinberger, J. (2003) *A Study of Family Support Work Conducted by Foxhill and Parson Cross Sure Start*. Sheffield: School of Education.

Chapter 19

Providing Respite for Parents

Brian Crosbie and Mark Avis

Family support covers a wide range of activities that stretch from early preventative interventions with vulnerable families to avert a crisis through to more intensive social support and provision of residential care in cases of family breakdown. The nature of family support offered within Sure Start Local Programmes was generally designed to provide flexible, targeted early interventions to avert family problems in the context of an overall programme intended to reduce social disadvantage (Glass 1999; Eisenstadt 2002). Two particular features of social disadvantage in some Sure Start areas is the parents' experience of social isolation and lack of support networks (Armstrong and Hill 2001; Cowen and Reed 2002). These circumstances can compound the problems faced by parents as they strive to be 'good enough' parents (Miller 2001, p.26), particularly when their socioeconomic situation does not allow them to pay for childcare when their ability to parent is challenged or becomes exhausted.

Respite scheme

A respite scheme was set out as part of the Radford/Hyson Green Sure Start Local Programme's initial delivery plan. The intention of the scheme was to provide responsive respite to families by offering flexible, time-limited childcare placements at local nurseries. Health or social care professionals in the Sure Start area could refer families who would benefit from respite by completing a referral form detailing the case for respite support. All referrals were reviewed by a Sure Start respite coordinator (health visitor and Sure Start Local Programme health lead), the allocation of respite was carried out at monthly meetings attended by the respite coordinator, and representatives from the local nurseries provided respite. In the three years the respite scheme was in operation up until November 2006, the scheme received 209 referrals and provided support to 129 children registered with Sure Start (an additional 80 children not registered with Sure Start were also awarded respite). The usual duration of respite was two sessions a week over four months, although some parents received more and others received only single sessions. In all, 6444 childcare attendances were recorded as a result of the scheme, with an average of 49 attendances for each child. At the monthly respite scheme meetings, professionals and nursery managers reviewed the ongoing needs of the children receiving respite.

Evaluation

The purpose of the evaluation was to provide a review of the scheme through the perceptions of parents who have used respite and the views of health and social care professionals, community workers and nursery managers who had referred families to respite care. The evaluation set out to explore the following four key objectives:

- to review referrals to respite care in order to identify the main reasons for referral and to describe use of the service

- to describe parents' experiences of respite care, with particular reference to the difficulties and benefits associated with receiving the service

- to describe health professionals' views of respite care after they had referred parents and children to the service

- to review the processes involved in the allocation of respite care.

Methods

The data for the evaluation were gathered using a mixed methods approach (Bowling 2002). The first phase involved a systematic audit of 100 randomly selected respite referral forms containing demographic information about the families, as well as details of professional assessments of families' needs. The audit data were collated using an Excel spreadsheet, and the reasons for respite were grouped into categories such as 'need for socialisation' or 'behaviour management issues'. The second phase of the evaluation involved 15 interviews with a range of stakeholders, including five parents who had used the respite service, seven professional workers who had referred families to respite, two nursery managers who provided respite, as well as an interview with the respite scheme coordinator. The interviews lasted between 20 minutes and one hour, and covered interviewees' experiences and views about respite provision. All interviewees gave informed consent to take part, and the interviews were recorded. A thematic qualitative analysis was used to identify the beliefs, values and social processes that influenced the use and outcomes of respite.

Findings

Referrals

Almost half of the referrals came from health visitors (45%) with a further 20 per cent coming from Sure Start family support workers; other referrals were from social workers, portage workers, Early Years coordinators, or maternity support workers. The two most common reasons given for referral to respite were 'mental health issues' and 'social isolation'. However, these factors were usually associated with other, more particular, circumstances such as domestic violence, housing issues, chronic illness, or parenting issues (such as behaviour management). Referrals also mentioned specific one-off circumstances such as a hospital appointment or access to a debt-counselling appointment, or instances where parents were studying or needed some time for themselves.

Referral forms also identified the child's need for respite, although these reasons usually reflected the circumstances of their parents. Parents' mental health problems or feelings of isolation were thought to have an influence on their confidence in meeting their child's development or socialisation needs. Furthermore, isolated parents were thought to be unlikely to seek support and guidance for these problems. Many of the referral forms also requested respite in order that parents could support and spend time with their other children.

The professionals we interviewed were clear that a need for respite could not be assessed on the basis of a standard measure that identified a family's need. As interviewees pointed out, offering respite should not be restricted to

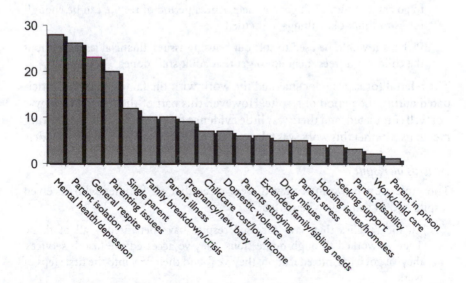

Figure 19.1 Reasons for referrals to respite (all reasons relating to parents given in 100 referral forms)

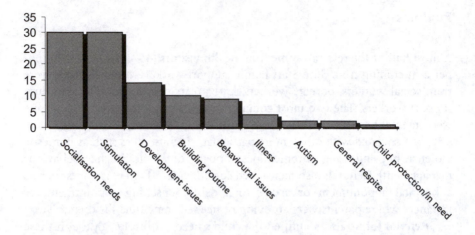

Figure 19.2 Reasons for referrals to respite (all reasons relating to children given in 100 referral forms)

families in crisis, and professionals placed great emphasis on using respite to pre-empt families falling into crisis or as a resource from which parents could increase their capacity through work or education. Professionals felt that they could use respite to respond to a wide variety of family needs.

> We can pre-empt the situation. Some time the parent states that they are going to go crazy if they can't get any help. And a period of respite can be enough for us to think okay things are settled.

> Perhaps it would be used to sort out housing issues, financial issues without the child. So it frees them up to get that adult stuff done.

The referral forms also documented the work with the family that was anticipated during the period of respite. However, this part of the referral form was not well completed, and there was little evidence from the monthly monitoring meetings whether this work was taking place or what progress had been made.

Benefits of respite

The professionals we interviewed were clear that all families who received respite had in some way benefited.

> All the families that have accessed respite have benefited – all of them. They've worked through depressions, they've accessed the health services, they've got back into education, they've found their way into the first steps of work

Interviews with parents and professionals identified some of the ways that parents and children had benefited from respite. We could recognise two main

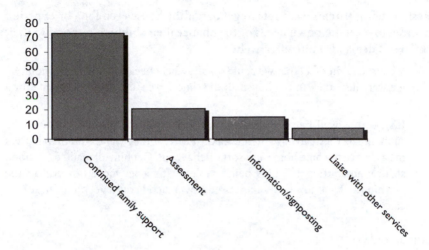

Figure 19.3 Work to be carried out with the family during respite as identified on 100 referral forms

ways in which families derived a benefit from respite: having a breathing space and building capacity.

BREATHING SPACE

A common theme for parents and professionals was a recognition of the way in which respite had allowed parents to have some time for themselves in order to reflect, recuperate or organise their lives. Parents drew attention to the importance of having some time for themselves or to recuperate from the demands of parenting.

> I feel a bit better in myself. I could feel down at times you know… I enjoyed the space without him so as I could get on with things. I couldn't cope with it all because I'm on anti-depressants because of all this. Now I feel a lot better in myself.

> Respite care helped me and my partner to catch up on the sleep that we missed, and to get things done. So it was like recharging me and my partner so we could cope when they came home from school. So we're not always tired and zombies.

> Quality time with my partner mainly: we don't get much time because of our kids. We were near to splitting up a few times.

The interviews with professionals and parents suggested that, for many parents, the inability to find time for a breathing space was associated with parents' feelings of isolation and loneliness. A lack of breathing space exacerbated their experience of isolation and could cause a further barrier to socialisation.

Respite meant parents were able to get out of the house even for a brief period in order to meet their own needs or to enhance their ability to respond to their children's demands more effectively.

> We just couldn't feel that we could go anywhere because of his behaviour. So we were just stuck in the house all the time…we were really desperate for a break.

> It's good as well because they can go at 7.30 in the morning, so if we're running late they can have their breakfast there if they want. And then it gives me a chance to come home and sort Michael out. Get him all ready for school, so he's not hitting the kids being violent. It's a lot more peaceful in the morning… I was just really impressed how much I could get out of it, sort of catch up.

BUILDING CAPACITY

All the parents we spoke to felt that respite had been a positive experience for their children, particularly in helping their children to develop social confidence.

> The nursery learns them things that I don't teach them. For one, they've got independence from their mum. I also think it has built their trust and security with other adults.

> He benefited quite a lot. He calmed down most ways. He enjoyed going. He behaved himself quite well in nursery. Not quite as much at home, but it was bad before he started there. But he did calm down quite a bit… It built his confidence and got him used to playing with children…he wouldn't play with anyone. And when he did mix, he was a bit violent towards them. Kicking, punches. But he got quite into the nursery, he calmed down he stopped doing those things. He doesn't do anything like that any more… I can manage it now.

Parents also noted improvements in their child's previous challenging behaviour, and acknowledged that nursery staff had helped their child to address problems that had been impossible to tackle at home. Parents also recognised that the developmental input offered by nurseries had addressed problems around learning deficits. With the continued support of nursery staff and others, this meant that they were able to deal with their children more effectively in the home.

> They told me they dealt with children who had violence in the family…and after a while he started to come on quite well in nursery.

Respite also provided an opportunity for parents take action about their own needs or address family issues affecting a child's development. Parents described how respite had given them the opportunity to seek advice concerning their own needs or to deal with their own mental health issues. Similarly, professionals described circumstances where respite was used proactively to support ongoing work with the family in order to avert further difficulties. These included debt counselling, housing support, and domestic violence support groups.

> It's made me a hell of a lot calmer and knowing that...there's no need to panic. There's somebody there who's going to take Mary for a while and I can have my time, which is important... I went on parenting things and behaviour management things and they really helped at a time when I really needed help.

> We give them a programme of work to do and with nursery nurse support it could be parenting issues, behaviour issues or phobia. Or they need help leaving the house, it could be that parents need to access other services like counselling service. So we offer respite so that the parent can attend these services.

REFLECTIONS ON RESPITE

Parents, professionals and nursery managers all stressed that a key feature of the benefits of the respite scheme was communication between nursery staff, parents and Sure Start. It was important in helping parents to deal with issues at home, and offered parents a level of reassurance when leaving their children at the nursery. It also meant that nurseries were able to initiate support and add to the ongoing support for parents.

> Yeah, every time I picked him up, we would sit down and have a chat about how he's got on... A lot of places treat the kids as a group. And at the nursery that he goes to they treat them as individuals. So if someone's got an individual need they'll concentrate on that need.

Nursery staff felt that they became more involved with the family, and since they also attended the monthly meetings where children's progress is discussed they were able to contribute to the overall support that parents received. However, a health visitor observed that the health visiting contribution to monitoring a family's progress at monthly meetings could have been enhanced.

> We could have more case reviews. We could go to the nursery and have some time with the parent and Sure Start and find out how it is going, we're not doing that. We used to have review time, which I thought was quite helpful, to tell perhaps the parent that it's time to move on soon. Let's look at some other agencies to move on to, but we don't do that now... We don't feel quite so involved with that, the assessment after four months. We'll communicate through phone or by letter but we don't have joint meetings. Whether that's going on between Sure Start and the nursery, I'm not sure.

It is worth noting that the respite scheme appeared to have overcome some of the worries that families might have about seeking help. As one parent commented:

> Some families might seem put off with it [respite] because they feel that if they say that they're not coping then all these other agencies will get involved; they'll get grassed up to social services. But they don't; you're going to them and saying you've got a problem and you need help, and they'll help you anyway. A lot of people are scared. Saying that they can't cope and thinking they'll get social services down their neck, but they're not.

On the whole, interviewees were realistic about the outcomes that could be achieved in the context of a limited period of respite but many were concerned about the effects at the end of a period of respite. As part of their ongoing work with parents, professionals were able to draw in the expertise of community-based agencies to tackle particular issues such as domestic violence, debt counselling and training. There was a widespread view that respite could be targeted to more families who were considered to have complex needs, and some workers argued that periods of respite ought to be used to benefit all families in the Sure Start area.

> As far as targeting goes, I think respite is a good thing in itself, and should be offered to more families.

> I feel respite care could be offered to a larger audience. I think there are a lot of parents who could be offered a longer-term support so they can go back to education…what happens is that they can get on to a course but not enough time to do coursework; they'll do part of a course and that takes them so much longer to get out of their level of deprivation if you like.

The view that there should be some form of 'universal' provision of respite in the form of more accessible childcare for younger aged children perhaps reflects the limited range of responses that professionals feel is available to them when working with families in deprived areas and where parents face a complex set of problems related to social disadvantage. This point was firmly stated by a health visitor during an interview:

> Respite is such a support network, and we have nothing else to offer them. Day care for children doesn't exist unless you pay.

Conclusion

The provision of respite childcare placements in local nurseries was viewed by parents and professionals as an opportunity for parents to have a breathing space. A breathing space gave parents a time away from the pressures of parenting which they used to reflect on issues facing them, recoup their energy, or meet their own needs. Parents and professionals provided examples of how respite had increased parents' capacity to parent, and they could identify direct benefits for the child in increasing his or her social confidence. Parents and professionals were able to use respite proactively to try and resolve problems such as debt and housing, attend groups, or to complete coursework for educational or vocational qualifications. Respite offers parents a breathing space that gives them the opportunity to be proactive rather than reacting to situations in their lives. It is a form of family support that can help parents out of 'crisis mode and into a capacity that will allow them to think about future development' (Wiggins *et al.* 2005, p.84).

Professionals involved in respite shared the view that respite held advantages for children who were otherwise experiencing levels of isolation detrimental to their well-being and acquisition of social skills, although they did voice concerns about the use of respite in responding to long-term issues confronting some families. Good communication between parents, nurseries and Sure Start staff was important in encouraging parents to feel secure about leaving their children in day care. Parents spoke of having positive and timely feedback on their child's progress and respite gave parents the opportunity to seek out advice on handling challenging behaviour in the home. Consequently, nurseries had been able to contribute to family support directly, helping parents to deal with problems at home and by providing advice and guidance on specific problems. However, documentation regarding children's progress was minimal, and this made it difficult to gather evidence from the referral process on the effectiveness of the respite provision.

There was general agreement that respite has a part to play in preventing vulnerable families from falling into a crisis which necessitates social service involvement (Appleton 1996; Carpenter, Griffiths and Brown 2005). The question of extending respite to more families within a Sure Start area would have to be weighed up against the arguments for retaining targeted respite for highly vulnerable families and children. This argument centres on available resources and the benefits of universal versus targeted provision of funded family support services in the context of the socioeconomically deprived areas covered by Sure Start (Elkan and Robinson 2001). However, as Appleton (1996) reports, the low-level interventions and amelioration of family strife of the kind offered by respite are difficult to capture in terms of current evaluation strategies (Elkan, Blair and Robinson 2000). Indeed, the benefits of early preventative interventions with vulnerable families to avert a crisis can be missed by an evaluation strategy that seeks to identify the longer-term fiscal advantages to government sectors such as education, criminal justice or adult health. The long-term benefits to families will come through strengthening support networks that enable parents to cope with family events and child behaviour issues before they become unmanageable.

Implications for Children's Centres

- Flexible, time-limited respite childcare is a useful means to avert crises developing within families and to provide a breathing space for parents under pressure. It can encourage parents to be proactive and children to gain benefits from their experiences in nursery.

- Respite schemes need to have robust systems for recording the work with the family to be carried out during respite which could be used to coordinate the input to families receiving respite.

- There is scope to include local nurseries more strategically in work with parents to develop parenting capacity and to help with children's specific needs.

References

Appleton, J.V. (1996) 'Working with vulnerable families: a health visitor perspective.' *Journal of Advanced Nursing 23*, 5, 912–918.

Armstrong, C. and Hill, M. (2001) 'Support services for vulnerable families with young children.' *Child and Family Social Work 6*, 4, 351–358.

Bowling, A. (2002) *Research Methods in Health: Investigating Health and Health Services.* Buckingham: Open University Press.

Carpenter, J., Griffiths, M. and Brown, S. (2005) *The Impact of Sure Start on Social Services.* Durham: Centre for Applied Social Research: The University of Durham.

Cowen, P. and Reed, D. (2002) 'Effects of respite care for children with developmental disabilities: evaluation of an intervention for at risk families.' *Public Health Nursing 19*, 4, 272–283.

Eisenstadt, N. (2002) 'Sure Start: key principles and ethos.' *Child Care, Health and Development 28*, 1, 3–4.

Elkan, R. and Robinson, J. (2001) 'Universal vs. selective services: the case of British health visiting.' *Journal of Advanced Nursing 33*, 1, 113–119.

Elkan, R., Blair, M. and Robinson, J. (2000) 'Evidence-based practice and health visiting: the need for theoretical underpinnings for evaluation.' *Journal of Advanced Nursing 31*, 6, 1316–1323.

Glass, N. (1999) 'Sure Start: the development of an early intervention programme for young children in the United Kingdom.' *Children & Society 13*, 4, 257–264.

Miller, S. (2001) 'Positive parenting: a sure start for children?' *Paediatric Nursing 13*, 9, 26–30.

Wiggins, M., Rosato, M., Austerberry, H., Sawtell, M. and Oliver, S. (2005) *Sure Start Plus National Evaluation: Final Report.* London: Social Science Research Unit, Institute of Education: University of London.

Chapter 20

What Difference Does Outreach Make to Family Support?

Brid Featherstone, Martin Manby and Nicky Nicholls

This chapter emerges from an evaluation of the work of an outreach team in one second-wave Sure Start programme. The evaluation attempted to capture the impact, as perceived by parents, of a range of interventions on parents' and children's health, confidence, social relationships and behaviour. Workers' perceptions on such issues, as well as broader observations on specific issues, were also explored. The chapter will outline the background to the programme, the evaluation and methods used, before exploring how the findings extend and contribute to discussions about the complexities of relationship building between workers and service users.

Doing it differently: the national background

In launching Sure Start, the then Secretary of State for Education, David Blunkett, spoke of wanting to do 'something that would be entirely new and innovative from the word go, to get to the core of the difficulties facing families and communities' (quoted in Gardner 2002, p.135). He argued that one of the key difficulties for service providers was the deep cynicism about professionalism, about government in all its guises, about agencies and departments. Sure Start was intended to be different from the start. For example, programmes were charged with reaching all residents within a specified geographical boundary (albeit within a restricted age range). This was to be a universal service designed alongside, and run in conjunction with, parents. The hope was that outward-reaching, locally designed and delivered services would not only counter cynicism, but would also reduce the distrust and fear of services, such as social service departments, as well as the historical stigma attached to help-seeking. This was, of course, quite complex in practice, given that it was a programme of centrally funded services attached to centrally set targets.

On the ground, however, Sure Start has been seen as a new and welcome beginning to provision of services for children and families by workers from a wide variety of both professional and non-professional backgrounds. As

Tunstill *et al.* (2005, p.164 [italics in original]) noted: 'In some ways the most important aspect of the SSLP (Sure Start Local Programme) is the stress on removing *barriers to access*, which have bedevilled the delivery of services for children and families over a very long period'. In this context, as members of the national evaluation team (NESS), Tunstill *et al.* suggest that of all the services delivered, outreach is crucial, not only in delivering such services successfully, but also in engaging the community, particularly those deemed 'hard-to-reach'.

The notion of 'hard-to-reach' is problematic and has been used differently at different points in Sure Start's history. It is often applied to categories of people, such as minority ethnic populations, lone mothers or fathers, as well as parents in full-time work. Indeed, it has appeared at times that vulnerability and/or need has been read off categorical status; at other times, 'hard-to-reach' has been used to denote a service deficit issue (for example, the timing of services may exclude fathers or those working). Whatever the many problems attached to the term, the attention and priority given to engaging the 'hard-to-reach' by policy makers and many programmes is important and interesting, and *is* a distinctive marker between Sure Start and other services, particularly social services departments, which have had to put a premium on gate-keeping and rationing demand for services.

Generally, the emergence of locality-based programmes, which are well resourced and explicitly designed to be universal in their reach, has expanded the knowledge base within family support. For example, Tunstill *et al.* (2005) suggest, from their evaluation of outreach services across programmes, that there are differing types of service users: autonomous, facilitated and conditional. Autonomous users are those who are keen and/or able to use services, provided they have the appropriate information available to them. The other two groups need more help and thus reinforce the potential importance of outreach teams, their principles and underpinning structures.

Sure Start Bramley: background and evaluation

The Sure Start initiative was announced in 1998 and trail blazer programmes were introduced in 1999. Second- and third-wave programmes followed, with Sure Start Bramley (SSB), a second-wave programme, gaining approval from the Sure Start Unit in 2000. The current evaluation team was appointed at the end of 2000. A subgroup for the evaluation was established, the membership of which has varied over the six years, but which has included parental involvement for much of this time. Whilst local evaluation teams have received guidance and support from regional and national Sure Start, and there have been some specific requirements in relation to their priorities, in general, it is the evaluation subgroup and the SSB management team who have agreed priorities which have been set annually. The remit for the specific piece of work discussed here emerged from this process.

The remit was to enable a detailed exploration of the views of families about the impact upon parents and children of the work carried out or organised by the outreach team. The outreach team comprises five workers and a manager, some of whom live locally, who come from a variety of backgrounds with varying professional qualifications, and carry specified caseloads assessed as requiring ongoing case management. Their work is embedded within a centre programme which includes parent information workers, play and development workers, and crèche workers.

It was agreed that the evaluation methodology would be mainly qualitative with parents being interviewed at a venue and time of their choice. However, the qualitative interviews were supplemented by completion of assessment grids which attached a numerical score to both 'impact', in a variety of domains, and parents' assessment of the contribution of SSB to this impact. Two grids were used, one focusing on parents and one on children.

The criterion for inclusion in the research was set at either a minimum of three months' contact or six home visits. The target number was initially 20–25 families, but in the event, successful interviews were completed with 18. Given the age range of the children catered for by SSB, it was agreed that they would not be interviewed. Although interview times were offered to cater for working patterns and, where appropriate, invitation letters were sent to both parents, in practice it was mothers who responded and volunteered for interview. In most cases, interviews were also held with the workers attached to the families. A focus group with the manager and three members of the team was also held after completion of the family interviews. Most interviews with parents, and the focus group with workers, were taped and transcribed. A thematic analysis of the qualitative data was undertaken and the scores attached to differing domains in the assessment grids calculated: the findings from these are the basis of this chapter.

This piece of research is part of a bigger picture in relation to evaluation of the work of the outreach team at SSB. Importantly, for the last three years, a file review has been undertaken which looks at the overall profile of work undertaken throughout the year and has provided a picture of the demographic features of clients, the kinds of problems referred, the key referral agents and the overall level of work undertaken by the team. The file review provided contextual data for this evaluation.

Findings

Demographic features: who, why and how long?

Two-thirds of the participants were lone mothers (12). This proportion is higher than in the general profile found in the file review. The majority described themselves as white British (14), with four being from minority ethnic groups. The area under review does not contain a significant minority ethnic population, although it does have a dispersal centre for asylum seekers which has been a focus for SSB work (one interviewee was an asylum seeker). Overall, family size, in terms of numbers of children, was higher than in the general population with half (nine) having three or more children.

Over half (ten) the participants appeared to have multiple needs and many were receiving, or had received, a wide variety of services. For example, one woman, who had been involved with the team since the inception of SSB, had sought and been provided with help in relation to: isolation, housing, depression, relationship with partner and family, information on child development and managing children's behaviour. Other services offered to other families included: transport to services, attendance at medical appointments, rubbish clearing, assistance with moving house, debt counselling, smoking cessation, playgroups, training courses, volunteering and taking part in trips. Services were accessed from Sure Start facilities, as well as via local organisations with service level agreements with the programme. Established working relationships with local statutory agencies were a feature of most of the cases. The average length of contact between these families and the team was about two years, which was much longer than that found in the file review, where the average length of contact was about six months.

Did things improve?

FINDINGS FROM THE GRIDS

Fourteen assessment grids were completed in relation to 16 children. The highest impact appeared to be on children's development (14/16 improved), followed by learning (13/16), and making new friends (13/16). Parents also reported positive impacts on children's speech and language (11/16) and confidence (11/16). Improved behaviour was observed for just over half the children (9/16). Less improvement was observed in children's health (3/16 with eight remaining the same). Where parents identified improvements, SSB was perceived as being the major contributory factor. To give just one example here, 12 children were scored as having improved in relation to making new friends, with SSB scored as the main contributory factor for all of them.

Seventeen grids were completed providing data on parents. The clearest gains were in relation to confidence (improved for 16/17), motivation (15/17) and isolation/contacts (14/17). The majority made new friends (14/17) and developed new parenting skills (13/17). Again, Sure Start involvement was seen as the main contributory factor to these improvements: all who reported their confidence, motivation or level of isolation had improved or much improved gave Sure Start the highest possible score as a contributory factor.

QUALITATIVE DATA

Whilst the grids provided much valuable information in relation to outcomes, the interviews with the mothers, and the subsequent discussions with workers, provided a rich pool of data, particularly in relation to process issues. A number of issues emerged about relationships between service users and individual workers, and between service users and the programme. Several themes were generated under this umbrella which relate to how workers and service users (the vast majority of whom were women) negotiated the interface between being friendly and being a friend, and anxieties about dependency which emerged in many of the cases. Light was also thrown on how workers, in their everyday practice, stayed and worked with the anxieties which emerged from remaining open and negotiating around dilemmas, rather than relying on rule-bound and rigid mechanisms, such as the strict use of timescales.

The fine line between being friendly and approachable and remaining professional was a theme running through the workers' focus group data. As one participant said: 'You've got to be very aware of professional boundaries'. This statement opened up a discussion which suggested that 'awareness of professional boundaries' was not a neat, once-and-for-all process, as the statement could imply, but involved ongoing, contextual negotiations which were linked to individual situations. For example, there was recognition that because some of the families had little contact with their own extended families, 'they see you as a friend', or sometimes as their substitute family. Data from the interviews showed that some service users certainly felt this way, especially if their parents were dead, or consistently hostile or disengaged, and/or they had difficulties of their own (e.g. alcoholism). Workers also recognised that, for some service users, their relationships with adult partners could either be non-existent, disappointing and/or violent. In these cases, a worker's involvement might have a reparative element to it, as in this example: 'Offering a hug to someone who hasn't been hugged for ages because they have not got a partner or whatever else'. One mother was seen as 'having had a lot of messy endings in her life', and therefore how time limits were used was seen as important by both the worker and the mother.

The theme of 'appropriate disclosure' also emerged in the focus group as potentially helpful with relationship building. Whilst there was evidence of adherence to a professional consensus that personal disclosure can destabilise professional boundaries, it was recognised that, in practice, this had to be tempered by the need for active, ongoing renegotiation of professional boundaries.

> I think we do give a bit of ourselves in a professional way. People don't know where we live. They don't know all about our lives, but I think because we do give a little bit sometimes…just to know that you've got a child does actually

help them...'cos they don't see you as somebody who's learnt it out of a text book.

As other evaluations of programmes highlight, and as the NESS evaluation repeats (Tunstill *et al.* 2005), *how* services are delivered and *how* workers engage service users is crucial. Communicating respect and using professional expertise in an accessible and sensitive way are central here. Our evaluation found clear evidence that all service users experienced the services provided as helpful and respectful, as these comments show.

> They gave me my respect and dignity... They keep the balance between helping and not invading my privacy... They praise me (and) tell me what I'm getting right.

> In the beginning, when I came here, I was almost feeling like crying. Talking to [N] she made me much stronger emotionally, and also mentally and physically... I have to say Bramley Sure Start, they give me very much some power inside of myself...to be very strong.

> It's so marvellous to wake up... You feel relieved because you can go there. It makes me happy.

THE FILE REVIEW

The file review conducted over the previous three years in SSB suggested that autonomous clients constitute the majority of those who engage with Sure Start. This piece of more intensive research suggests that the other groupings identified by Tunstill *et al.* (2005) are evident, but the categories are less discretely constituted than they suggest. For example, we found instances throughout the sample of the value of flexibly combining practical and therapeutic services for a variety of service users and, moreover, that service users' needs were linked to changing levels of need, or changing circumstances, rather than operating in a linear way according to a mythical 'type' of user. A clear finding from all the data gathered with workers and service users was that SSB, as a well-resourced programme, was able to deploy services in a flexible way, according to changing needs and circumstances, rather than fit service users into pre-existing programmes, or move them along in a pre-determined way. This again marks Sure Start out as distinctive and is partly why the shift to Children's Centres has been so anxiety-provoking for many workers, as resources will be spread much more thinly, with family support-type services appearing particularly vulnerable.

In the next section we offer some thoughts from our evaluation which we consider contribute to contemporary discussions about the challenges and opportunities in delivering such a valued service.

Making a difference

All workers articulated a sense that handling the professional/friend dichotomy was messy and uncomfortable at times. They used a range of formal and informal mechanisms, including supervision and offloading to other team members, to talk through dilemmas (i.e. being friendly and accessible and not offering false hopes to service users about being available as a friend). It was clear that the formal and informal organisational climate which had been established was vital in terms of offering opportunities to talk through issues, encourage humour and, most importantly, learn from each other. (For wider discussion on organisational climate and culture, see Hall 1999.)

The interlinked question of 'dependency' was raised by both workers and service users. The term, generally and in policy and practice terms, has had pejorative connotations. Currently, in policy terms, the presumption is that attaining independence through involvement in paid work is the desired outcome for adults and, indeed, Sure Start programmes have been promoted as part of this policy drive. However, the importance of recognising, celebrating and positively facilitating our *interdependence*, rather than valorising independence, is increasingly stressed by those critical of current policy directions (Williams 1999). Our limited findings suggest that the workers and service users we encountered had developed practices which neither denied dependency as a feature of relationships, nor managed it by a rigid one-size-fits-all system (such as structured time limits for services or rigid referral protocols). Moreover, this may be of interest in the context of developments within the literature on family support, suggesting that for families with interlocking and ongoing difficulties, which may be historically entrenched, it may be valuable to engage with concepts such as 'managed dependency' where, for example, there are no rigid cut-off points for service provision (Turney 2005).

The interviews with service users suggest that 'dependency' had been the subject of considerable discussion between them and individual workers. Although not always resolved to the satisfaction of everyone, either in terms of meanings or practices, the overwhelmingly positive feedback received from service users about individual workers, and the service overall, suggests that an open, dialogical approach may be more respectful than, for example, using procedural means to manage difficult feelings. This is all the more interesting in the light of the evidence that time limits were not used in a strict or rigid way by workers to manage encounters.

To conclude this section, whilst the evaluation focused on the work of one team, the team was embedded within a centre and a programme. It is important to note that we observed and received considerable feedback on how important other staff were, from the reception staff onwards (indeed, particularly the reception staff as the initial 'face' of the programme). One woman who had been cut off from her own parents by her abusive husband described Sure Start as: 'Very welcoming…like a big happy family'.

Conclusion

This chapter provides a snapshot of an aspect of one programme. It suggests that for the service users who took part in the evaluation, considerable improvements in their lives had occurred and that, moreover, working practices had been developed and sustained which were experienced as both helpful and respectful. A wide menu of services was available and offered by well-resourced workers in a flexible and individualised way. It remains to be seen, however, whether the planned, less well-resourced shift to Children's Centres will be able to sustain these gains.

Implications for Children's Centres

- Clarity is needed in relationship building between professionals and parents in the context of new, more informal, 'befriending' ways of working and interacting.

- Dependency within relationships needs to be recognised and managed in an open manner.

References

Gardner, R. (2002) *Supporting Families: Protecting Children in the Community.* Chichester: Wiley/NSPCC.

Hall, C. (1999) 'Integrating services for children and families: the way forward.' *Children and Society 13,* 3, 216–222.

Tunstill, J., Allnock, D., Akhurst, S., Garbers, C. and the Ness Research Team (2005) 'Sure Start Local Programmes: implications of case study data from the National Evaluation of Sure Start.' *Children and Society 19,* 2, 158–172.

Turney, D. (2005) 'Who cares? The role of mothers in cases of child neglect.' In J. Taylor and B. Daniel (eds) *Child Neglect: Practice Issues for Health and Social Care.* London: Jessica Kingsley.

Williams, F. (1999) 'Good enough principles for welfare.' *Journal of Social Policy 28,* 4, 667–689.

Chapter 21

Enaging with Men

Lynne McKenna

In the course of evaluating a number of local Sure Start projects, the involve-ment of men emerged as a recurring imperative. The projects all stated their intent to increase the involvement of fathers in the physical, intellectual and social development of babies and young children, and expressed expectation of increasing male involvement in wider activities. Sure Start practice guidance reinforces this: 'All Sure Start Children's Centre services should be responsive to the level of local need to support fathers in their relationship with their partner and in their role as a parent' (Sure Start 2005, p.54).

However, the ways in which projects attempted to do this varied across the programmes. From practitioners' interviews it emerged that, for some, Sure Start was seen as the provision of a set of activities. According to this image, success was associated with registering the attendance of men at activities. To assume, therefore, that because men were not participating in courses, or involved in meetings, means that projects are not reaching out to men is too simplistic. This chapter explores the ways in which the various levels of father involvement are actually making a positive contribution to the physical, intel-lectual and social development of young children.

The New Town Sure Start fathers' group has been meeting at the local community centre on Sunday mornings for the past three years. A community development worker with responsibility for encouraging fathers facilitates this group. Sunday mornings have proved successful in recruiting and retaining fathers for this group, and currently nine fathers and 22 children attend on a regular basis.

However, rather than simply counting fathers' involvement as attendance at Sure Start activities, New Town Sure Start has been working towards supporting fathers in their relationships with their children, developing per-ceptions of themselves as parents, and the development of 'fathering' skills as opposed to 'mothering' skills. While wider participation within Sure Start, and indeed the community itself, has been encouraged, this has often been the result of a 'spin off' rather than an objective.

The literature reveals that this planned approach is not widespread among such programmes. Ghate, Shaw and Hazel (2000), investigating family centres, found that centres were more concerned about having an identifiable strategy for working with fathers than the rationale behind that strategy. Meyers (1993) noted that because there have been few studies on fathers with regard to their participation within the family and in childcare projects, community initiatives have little research to enlighten them about how to proceed. Whilst trying to encourage fathers to participate in the work of Sure Start projects, and in family life at home, we still have a very vague idea of what kinds of things might be helpful for fathers to participate in, why they might want to participate, and whether participation might have any beneficial effect on their family life.

Changing notions of fatherhood

Statistics from the National Parenting Family Institute (O'Brien 2004) reveal that UK men work the longest hours in Europe, an average of 48 hours a week for those with children under 11. While studies have shown that many fathers do now spend more time caring for their children, according to this evaluation, mothers are still the ones who spend the most time with them. However, research into involvement tends to be research into predominantly female environments and activities, with the father's role valued against a framework of activities identified with mothering.

Research has suggested that fathers' involvement supports the life chances of their children. Indeed, positive father involvement in children's learning is associated with better educational, social and emotional outcomes for children (Department for Education and Skills 2004; Flouri, Buchanan and Bream 2002; Goldman 2004). Similarly, children with involved fathers appear to avoid high-risk behaviours, compared to children who have uninvolved fathers (Horn and Sylvester 2002).

Methods

This research was conducted over an 18-month period and included semistructured interviews undertaken with the Sure Start programme manager and the community development worker. I visited the group on several occasions, initially to introduce myself informally to the fathers and children, and to begin data collection. A focus group discussion was held with the attending fathers in January 2005, followed by eight semistructured interviews conducted with individual fathers during March and April 2005, and February and March 2006. These interviews were followed up by a further focus group which was held in March 2006, as the culmination of one and a half years' full involvement in the group, to consider the longer-term impact on father–child relationships, the development of fathering skills and fathers' levels of participation within New Town Sure Start.

Findings and discussion

The research revealed that fathers' involvement in both their children's lives and, indeed, in Sure Start activities, appeared to be concerned with three main issues: confidence, challenging traditional views of fatherhood, and 'being there'.

The fathers in the New Town Sure Start talked about developing their confidence in being a father. This necessarily involved this group of fathers challenging traditional views of fatherhood, based on their own experience of being fathered, and subsequently becoming fathers themselves. Finally, one of the key findings to emerge from this research was the fathers' acknowledgement of their own need to 'be there' for their children.

Key issues

CONFIDENCE

One of the fathers interviewed discussed how his daughter was the first New Town Sure Start baby, and how his involvement in the group had enabled him to develop his ability as a new father. Being with other men had given this father a forum to share his uncertainties about his skills as a father of a new baby. The other men had been supportive, and he remarked on how the men had laughed at the way in which women thought themselves to be experts on babies and young children. A view was expressed that mothers often exert control over the family and not only decide whether their partner's involvement is or is not required, but feel secure enough in their mothering skills to make judgements on the quality of such involvement.

Lamb (1986) maintains that the development of self-confidence is a key factor which determines how fathers become involved with their children. Once fathers realise children are fun, Lamb believes that they should be able to expand the activity context.

I observed a father as he followed his 16-month daughter around the centre while she explored toys. When an older child offered to 'look after the baby', the father said: 'Just leave her. If she falls, she'll learn'. He described how his daughter had had to be taken to hospital during the previous week as she had fallen and bruised her forehead. He explained how having had experience of two children had helped him to remain calm and feel more confident in such situations.

One father discussed how his involvement in the fathers' group had allowed him to spend more time with his children. He explained that when he came in from work, his children were often off doing other things. The Sunday morning group had allowed him time to spend with his children and this, in turn, had stopped both his wife and his children complaining that he did not spend enough time with them. This father expressed satisfaction in the development of his skills as a parent, but more specifically in the development of his self-confidence as a father.

This idea of confidence in fathering is one which emerged in many discussions with the fathers. As one father explained: 'I sometimes get frustrated with the kids, but I try to talk to them and sort the problem out'. Another father thought attendance at the group had contributed to his perception of himself as a parent and claimed: 'I'm just as important as their mam!'

CHALLENGING TRADITIONAL VIEWS OF FATHERING

Despite the increasingly 'hands-on' reality of fathering for many men, cultural stereotypes of fathers as 'providers' and 'breadwinners' continue to exert a strong influence over men, women and children's attitudes to parenthood.

However, one father discussed how when men usually talk about their children (for example, at work or in the pub), children are often referred to in terms of what they have done wrong (e.g. disturbing their father's night). This father's involvement in the group had enabled him and the other fathers to develop an ongoing discourse that centred on their children's developing abilities, rather than presenting problems. This was illustrated as two fathers watched a two-year-old girl complete a jigsaw. They began to discuss whether this was advanced behaviour for such a young child. Comparisons were drawn between other children, and the men concluded that this young child was indeed advanced. The father of the child in question went on to discuss how having the opportunity to observe his children play enabled him to learn more about their interests and development.

The way in which men traditionally discussed their children was challenged by this group. The 'deficit' view of being a father was being replaced with a more balanced view, where it was acceptable to discuss the positive aspects of fathering, such as pride in their children's achievements. The fact that the men relished this opportunity reflects the way in which notions of fatherhood are changing. Traditionally considered to be a mother-type conversation, opportunities to discuss their children's development and progress were given a forum within this group.

During another visit to the Sunday morning group, three fathers watched as their older children played a board game. The fathers discussed the ways in which the children were quickly becoming experts at playing this game, as they were gaining more experience each week. The conversation then centred on the ways in which their children were developing certain skills as they played the game. One father expressed his pride that his child was able to 'take turns' in the game. Another father commented on his son's acquisition of number language as he counted spaces to be moved forward or backwards. The fathers discussed the educational potential of such board games and one father said:

> You would never think they could learn so much from playing a simple game. Having the time to sit back and watch and try to understand what is going on in their minds is a wonderful opportunity. It's something I never have time to do at home.

The fathers' rationale for being part of the group also emerged during discussions. One father recounted how his involvement had impacted upon his son's social development. This child had at first been very reluctant to leave his father's side but was now confidently wandering off and playing with other children. This father also considered that their involvement in the group had contributed to his son's language development. Although not claiming that the group was totally responsible for these two developments, this father was obviously proud that his involvement had influenced his son's development and enhanced their relationship. This evidence, from both interview and observation, is reflected in recent research which has shown that fathers who devoted time to their sons, even as little as five minutes a day, were giving them an enhanced opportunity to grow into confident adults (Buchanan and McCoy 1999).

One father interviewed identified that his children appeared better behaved when he was around. He wondered if this was down to the stereotypical approach his partner adopted when his children misbehaved: 'She uses me as a threat when they're naughty. She tells them, "You do that again and I'll tell your dad!" My mam used to do the same. She used to say "Wait till your dad gets in!"'

One of the discussions with the fathers revealed their perceptions of their fathering style compared to their own fathers. Three fathers discussed memories of their own childhood and their relationships with their own fathers. One father explained how his father had been a good role model and had been very involved in his upbringing. The other two fathers discussed not remembering their dads being involved until they were 14: 'I've only recently started actually talking to my dad. We have never fallen out or anything like that; we just had nothing to say to each other'.

The other father discussed how a dialogue with his own father had opened up for him since the birth of his own children.

> My dad hardly had anything to do with me but when we had the girls, he changed. It's all so different now. He drops everything when we ask him if he can look after them. It's the future I'm thinking of, I want my kids to look back and know I was there for them.

This was an interesting development for the group. As the fathers were talking about their own 'fathering' styles, many of them compared their own experiences from their childhood and examined their relationships with their own fathers. One father said: 'I have more time to spend with my kids than my dad ever did'.

BEING THERE

This notion of 'being there' was explored further as the fathers discussed being able to pick their children up from school on occasions as a privilege.

> I can't ever remember my dad picking me up from school. Sometimes when I pick them up and they moan all the way home about their day or the cold, I have to remind myself that it is great being able to pick them up.

One father who regularly picked his children up from school, but whose shift patterns at work were about to be changed, discussed how he intended to challenge his employers about 'family friendly' working practices. He discussed the importance of being able to be involved in his children's lives. As well as empowering these men to become more involved in their children's lives, it could be claimed that the discussions held in the group enabled dads to consider the level of involvement they wanted from their family life.

Spending time alone with their children was a theme which was discussed by most of the men in the focus group. One father discussed how the fathers' group allowed him two hours of unbroken time with his children.

> When the wife's around, I'm terrible. I tend to fall asleep or read a book or something. When I come here, I am in charge and it's great. It makes you feel better that you are spending time with your children. It's the same feeling you get when you've been to church. You feel good but you can't really explain why.

Fathers' levels of participation within New Town Sure Start

Many Sure Start projects appear to have at least one male who is an active contributor. However, the majority of men engaged in activities at New Town Sure Start are, at best, partakers of services.

One father who described himself as a 'behind the scenes contributor' was actively involved in planning events for the dads and worked closely with the community development worker. Early in this evaluation, this father had put forward his ideas about the way in which activities designed for men without children present would encourage the dads to interact and might actually benefit relationships in the longer term: 'Something like football or a gym or e-mail, or if we could buy some PlayStations – this would attract more men and older kids'. A successful bid to a local community foundation resulted in the group being able to purchase televisions and electronic games consoles as a resource for the older children of the group. Another father interviewed explained how these ideas would benefit the group.

> It's also good as it'll keep us up to speed with our children in terms of computer technology. We're not going to be left behind. It'll also give the kids whose parents can't afford PlayStations the opportunity. In the same way, it'll allow parents to ration time playing computer games.

Interestingly, the fathers questioned all discussed their partners' levels of participation. One father explained how his wife was a member of the management committee of New Town Sure Start and had been involved in another local Sure Start programme before moving to the area. As a 'serial Sure Start attender' his wife was positive about the benefits of her involvement. This father raised some interesting issues around his wife's involvement. He discussed how in his case this had resulted in a practical exchange of skills that has led to him spending more time with his children: 'She's come in from her course and has asked me to make playdough and all of us have played together. I have learnt from her. She passes it on'. From discussions, it was evident that, for some men, women's participation in a project had made a difference to the way they engaged with the family unit and with children: 'I am closer to the kids now 'cos she goes out. With the younger ones I watch them. I like looking after the kids. I didn't do that with the older ones 'cos she was always there for them'. This clearly shows that fathers were very interested in and, indeed, proud of their partners' involvement in Sure Start activities, but were content to keep their own involvement within the boundaries of the group and did not feel the need to extend their involvement to other Sure Start activities at this time.

One father explained that, while he would be interested in wider involvement in Sure Start, he was unable to come to some of the activities 'because most of the stuff that's on is on during the day'. As much of what happens in Sure Start projects is daytime activity, working men are often unable to attend. Given the high levels of unemployment in this Sure Start area, however, this does not appear to account for the exceptionally low level of involvement. One father revealed that he would feel uncomfortable coming to another Sure Start activity that was not specifically dedicated to men and children. The men generally said they felt uncomfortable about coming to courses mainly attended by women. Men suggested that activities on offer did not interest them as they were not aimed at developing their skills and knowledge.

The men I interviewed also complained that information is not sent out to the male member of the family and this means they are often unaware of what is going on in the centres and projects. One man stated: 'I would like to find out more and have all the information, as my partner only passes on what she wants', while another explained that it was not only getting the information, but seeing that information as being *meant for you*. One father noted that: 'Men are neglected from pregnancy in that mothers get books and information packs and all fathers get are leaflets'.

When asked how the group could attract more men from the local community, the fathers became quite animated. One father explained that being involved in the Sure Start fathers' group had heightened his awareness of the importance of being involved in his children's lives. This conversation sparked off a series of suggestions from the dads about future activities for the group.

A summer bike ride, cooking classes and outside visits were suggested. This illustrates the ways in which the community development worker is supporting the fathers to develop and take responsibility for this group. Lloyd, O'Brien and Lewis (2004) found that the presence of a dedicated member of staff to support fathers was a successful strategy for increasing father involvement.

Raikes *et al.* (2002) identified five stages of father involvement. In stages one and two, father involvement was not a priority. At stage three, a designated father involvement coordinator was appointed who promoted father involvement. At stages four and five, the programmes matured and supported fathers, both as parents and in their personal development, employing a father coordinator with specific training about father involvement.

This group is clearly at stage four on Raikes' involvement scale. The community development worker discussed how she had read about a free plastering course for men in the local newspaper. She asked the fathers if they would be interested, and secured places for two men on the course, which was run by a local trust. Similarly, a successful bid for a £2500 adult learning grant resulted in a free 26-week karate course for families, which attracted 17 families.

However, Meyerhoff (1994) urges caution about making a conscious effort to involve fathers. He suggests being more accepting of the contribution fathers actually do make. This research has illustrated the ways in which New Town Sure Start is doing just that.

We need to continue to ask questions about the role of men within a changing society, and whether getting men to attend centres might be denying the role men already play in parenting. By registering attendance at activities, could we be confusing the visible involvement of fathers in Early Years projects with effective involvement of fathers in their children's development? In spite of the plethora of books on child development and parenting, most women still learn most of what they know and believe from other women. Hitherto, most men have not been in regular social situations that encourage this kind of sharing of ideas about children's development. This group is one such social situation and may, therefore, have more importance and a wider impact than might be imagined. Local Sure Start programmes which *are* successful in the involvement of fathers perhaps need to consider ways in which they can disseminate and share successes and further promote the involvement of men. The work/life balance debate, and practices which have subsequently changed, have largely been conducted in terms of women as mothers. Only when the debate and policies are broadened to include men will there be a real possibility of them extending their family roles. There are major cultural and social obstacles that will need to be overcome before fathers can be fully included in mainstream family services that have traditionally been targeted at and used by mothers. Further research needs to be undertaken which differentiates between male and female as opposed to using the generic term 'parent'. There needs to be more explicit research into the nature of male involvement in projects and how this might be of value in improving family life and future opportunities for young children. Little research appears to have been done into fathering in its widest sense. Similarly, there appears to be little discussion, at a national level, about what policy makers and service providers can actually do to support men's parenting. This research has shown that although projects have been encouraged not to offer stereotypical activities for men, the men in this study have, so far, indicated that this is exactly what they want. Similarly, the idea that Sure Start projects should not rely on men's groups as the only activity catering to men, as they do not have universal appeal, is questioned by these findings. Interviews with this small group of men have revealed that it is only at such an activity that the men feel comfortable to make use of this service. It may be that traditionally male activities are essential as a first step for the majority of men.

Implications for Children's Centres

- There needs to be further work on disseminating and sharing good practice on involving men in Children's Centre activities.

- Further work is needed into evaluation of practices that support men's involvement in parenting.

- Increasing the involvement of men in Children's Centres and supporting men's parenting may require targeting their involvement at recognisable male activities where men feel more comfortable.

References

Buchanan, A. and McCoy, A. (1999) *Tomorrow's Men Project*. A Young Voice and Oxford University Project. Report available from adriennekatz@btinternet.com

Department for Education and Skills (2004) *Engaging Fathers, Involving Parents, Raising Achievement*. London: DfES.

Flouri, E., Buchanan, A. and Bream, V. (2002) 'Adolescents' perceptions of their fathers' involvement: significance to school attitudes.' *Psychology in the Schools 39*, 5, 575–582.

Ghate, D., Shaw, C. and Hazel, N. (2000) *How Family Centres are Working with Fathers Findings: Social Policy Research*. March 2000. Published by Joseph Rowntree Foundation and available at: www.jrf.org.uk/knowledge/findings/socialpolicy/330.asp, accessed on 23 August 2007.

Goldman, R. (2004) *Fathers' Involvement in Children's Education: a Review of the Research and Practice*. London: National Family and Parenting Institute.

Horn, W.F. and Sylvester, T. (2002) *Father Facts* (4th edition). Gaithersburg, MD: National Fatherhood Initiative.

Lamb, M.E. (1986) 'The changing role of fathers.' In M.E. Lamb (ed.) *The Father's Role: Applied Perspectives*. New York, NY: Wiley.

Lloyd, N., O'Brien, M. and Lewis, C. (2004) *Fathers in Sure Start*. London: University of London Institute for the study of Children, Families and Social Issues.

Meyerhoff, M.K. (1994) 'Of baseball and babies: are you unconsciously discouraging father involvement in infant care?' *Young Children May 1994*, 17–19.

Meyers, S. (1993) 'Adapting parent education programs to meet the needs of fathers: an ecological perspective.' *Family Relations 42*, 4, 447–463.

O'Brien, M. (2004) *Fathers and Family Support: Promoting Involvement and Evaluating Impact.* London: National Family and Parenting Institute.

Raikes, H., Boller, K., VanKemmen, W., Summers, J., Raikes, A., Laidble, D., Wilcox, B., Ontai, L. and Christensen, L. (2002) *Father Involvement in Early Head Start Programmes: a Practitioners' Study.* Princeton, NJ: Mathematical Policy Research.

Sure Start (2005) *Sure Start Children's Centres: Practice Guidance.* London: Sure Start.

Chapter 22

Issues in Evaluating Family Support Services

Anne Barton, Jill Jesson and Matthew Horton

The Family Support Service (FSS) in Sure Start Local Programmes (SSLPs) was a core service which focused on new approaches to working with families in both preventative and supportive ways. In recognition of their success, guidance for Sure Start Children's Centres emphasises that the core offer should include family support and outreach for parents.

In this chapter, we present some lessons learned from a review of the literature and a case study evaluation of one SSLP Family Support Service. The purpose is to draw out some of the aspects of FSS, which are generalisable, and to consider the implications for a future evidence-based service.

Family support services offered a new model of working by providing supportive, befriending, preventative work with families, which would be additional to services already provided by any existing organisations. Typically, family support staff worked in the community alongside families, providing something different from statutory agencies and childcare professionals. Some projects were built on existing family support services already set up by the voluntary sector (such as National Children's Homes, Action for Children or Home Start), which evolved along a number of routes following the Children Act 1989, and from social services and Early Years services. Most FSS had close links with health visitors and midwives, since they were the main path for recruitment of parents and children to Sure Start programmes. Others had close links to social and prevention services.

Study approach

The chapter is based on an evaluation of FSS which was completed in 2006. First of all, we wanted to find out how other programmes had evaluated their FSS. We posed the questions:

1. What theory or models underpinned FSS?

2. What were the key learning points from earlier evaluations?

3. What could we add to the knowledge base with our own evaluation?

4. How could we best meet the development needs of the client?

The first part of the chapter is based on an assessment of the published litera-ture, based on a general electronic search in 2005 of the National Evaluation of Sure Start (NESS) website (www.ness.bbk.ac.uk), which contains many of the SSLP evaluation reports. The search identified 12 reports. The main limitation of the electronic approach and the NESS website is that there may be other excellent FSS evaluation reports which we have not identified because they may be listed under another category, or embedded within other reports.

The second part of the chapter describes a case study evaluation under-taken by the authors (Barton *et al.* 2006).

What is family support?

The National Society for the Prevention of Cruelty to Children (NSPCC) noted that 'family support is a generic term covering an enormous number and diver-sity of activities meeting a comparable diversity of needs' (Gardner 2003, p.1). Generally speaking, FSS tend to have four guiding principles:

1. to identify and promote strengths in families and family members

2. to be explicitly or implicitly preventative in purpose

3. to emphasise solutions and mutual responsibility

4. to be community-based and voluntary.

The implicit simple values are that the FSS should be:

1. comprehensive

2. flexible

3. collaborative

4. family-centred.

From the 12 reports accessed from the NESS website it was possible to catego-rise three waves of FSS evaluation, each reflecting the stage of development of the Sure Start intervention. Early reports, dated 2001–2003, were mainly descriptive, covering the process of setting up the service. From 2003 to 2005, when services were up and running, reports attempted to quantify simple outputs and outcomes, such as describing the types of support provided and measuring user satisfaction. The third wave of reports (which would include our evaluations) explored issues of sustainability and additionality (e.g. assess-ing cost-effectiveness). They attempted to demonstrate tangible outcomes to provide evidence of impact.

Evaluating FSS poses challenges for evaluators. The philosophy or explicit value system is clear. Whilst models of family support share some core values (family-centred, flexible and collaborative), there is no single definition of a family support service. Some have their origins in health, some in social services, others in community development. This diversity of perspective means that services manifest themselves in different ways. We noted that very few FSS clearly defined their aims and objectives, and none of the evaluation reports defined what was meant by effectiveness of the service.

In addition, there were few reliable and robust measures of impact or effectiveness from which to draw evaluative conclusions. For instance, there was no quantification of the total number of cases and types of support provided over the life of the programme. It follows, therefore, that with weak data on demand for and use of resources it is difficult to demonstrate the cost-effectiveness of the service and the additionality delivered. To summarise the review, it was difficult to decide precisely what the FSS is because there was no single, robust definition of either the service or family support worker (FSW). It was equally unclear exactly what the service goals or outcomes would be.

It follows then that if the definitional boundary is conceptually loosely defined, and services tailored to family needs, variations and different manifestations of family support and the family support worker will occur. This variability across programmes made it difficult to make direct meaningful comparisons.

Comparison of other Sure Start Local Programme Family Support Services

The variability in the SSLP reports means that projects and outputs are not strictly comparable because they do not provide similar detail or information.

Experience showed that it often took up to three years for SSLPs to establish themselves, find a community-based building, recruit appropriate staff, involve the local community and then achieve a full range of functioning services. Many early FSS evaluations were undertaken in this early developmental phase. They were exploratory rather than evaluative, describing the procedures of developing a new service, and thus one might call them formative evaluations. Most evaluations assessed simple outcomes, such as levels of satisfaction of clients and perceptions of FSS staff or other statutory providers. So they provided insight for new FSS setting up a service in later rounds. They are positive and show the FSS as a successful initiative.

However, as noted earlier, many did not include enough detail from which to draw robust conclusions. They did not provide the detail we were looking for, such as information about case process, case management and workload, types of casework encountered, or give details of the length of time given to cases – in short, helping us to understand what works, where, for whom and under what conditions.

There are few reliable, robust, accepted measures which can show the impact of the core values and ideals on the well-being of children, families or communities. Interestingly, the consultants evaluating Sure Start Easton (Roberts and Man 2004) stated that they were not able to get a clear description of the service through workshop or written material. We note that not one of the early evaluation reports identified specified measurable outputs or outcomes, except an assessment against the five Sure Start core objectives.

In the next section we discuss some features of the evaluation reports, and focus on our attempt to define the model.

What have we learnt from other evaluation studies?

1. All the projects reviewed are physically located in their community. They offer one-to-one casework, be it long- or short-term contact, centre-based and outreach home visits to families.

2. All have set up group activities, with varying degrees of success.

3. Most units are small, from two to eight staff, depending on the programme. Staff are usually female, with a background in child education, nursing or social services.

4. The basis of activity varies depending on the model: for some it is prevention (for instance keeping children off the at-risk register), health promotion (not illness care), or meeting the social, emotional or spiritual needs of families.

5. The demands on the support worker are wide: case management, giving information, referral to other agencies, parent support and education. The range of knowledge needed is wide: health, education, child development, adult employment and recreational activities.

In addition to casework, all FSS arranged many group activities and tried to engage the 'hard-to-reach'. The FSS themselves concluded that local parents were not too keen on group activities; they struggled to engage young parents, fathers, and Black and minority ethnic (BME) families. In addition, our review gave pointers to future development and management concerns, when Children's Centres took over in 2006. Most of this centred on organisational outputs such as how many staff for how many hours, which group sessions are offered, and so on. Few considered mainstreaming issues, or offered examples of best practice or even good practice.

Models

We noted earlier that there are principally three models underpinning FSS: health-focused, social services-focused, or with community development origins. At operational level, delivery depends on the particular model chosen by each FSS. For example, Sure Start Easton (Roberts and Man 2004, p.2) lacks a precise definition of family support, but it is a good example of trying to capture exactly what FSS does: 'Family support provides registered parents with an opportunity to receive help on almost any issue that arises in their lives and can be assisted through a supportive hand and careful direction to relevant agencies'. The core feature is its uniqueness (Roberts and Man 2004, p.3): 'It is a different style of delivery. It does not replicate any other service being provided, although operational structure resembles a health visitor or health link worker, and occasionally areas of health may be advised on by a FSW'.

So the Easton 'model' could be described as *health-focused*. Similarly, Sure Start programmes in Sandwell have a FSS which is purely antenatal and postnatal home-visiting. Sandwell has a high perinatal mortality rate (Outreach Officer 2004). In this case there has been a mainstream FSW since 1989, through which paraprofessionals, trained in health promotion work, visit families to provide practical and emotional ante- and postnatal support. What the Sure Start FSS added was more time to listen, to develop closer inter-agency work, and provide practical support for parents.

By comparison, Sure Start Foxhill and Parson's model is based on a social services prevention outcome (Weinberger 2003, p.1). This model sets out: 'To identify and support vulnerable families, engage the hard-to-reach and work with existing agencies, especially preventing children being taken into care, or re-registered on the Child Protection Register'.

A third 'model' is practised by Sure Start Loxford (Cordis Bright 2004, p.6). This has no defined origin but its four stated objectives are:

- to encourage children's and clients' emotional and cognitive development
- to advise parents and carers on child development issues, e.g. breastfeeding
- to give practical advice and signposting to parents as needed
- to provide practical support to parents and carers.

However, whilst we were engaged in external evaluation of other SSLPs, we identified some 'grey literature' that was unpublished. This work had been carried out by internal evaluators for service review. Typically it addressed simple outcome measures. Within programmes, staff were beginning to categorise the types of problem encountered from closed case files and to document case vignettes. Their analysis shows that the FSW took on many problems outside the remit of health or social services professionals. This 'grey literature' provides the evidence-base that FSS workers met a previously unmet need, offering welfare advice advocacy.

Case study: Eight Village Sure Start model of family support

Our case study is an example of the third phase FSS evaluation, a Round 5 programme in the West Midlands. The discussion is based on two documents: the internal review of a sample of 32 closed case studies (Horton 2005), and the external evaluation of the FSS (Barton *et al.* 2006).

Our evaluation questions were:

1. Is there a clearly defined purpose for the FSS? If yes, is it meeting that purpose?

2. Does it have a declared aim, objectives, targets, and intended outcomes? If yes, are these variables measured and SMART (specific, measurable, achievable, realistic and time-bound)?

3. Is the FSS additional to mainstream services or is it duplicating services?

4. Is the FSS providing good quality services that parents use, value and like?

Although a core component of Sure Start philosophy included family support, the real need for a local FSS was confirmed following parent consultation, which was undertaken to inform the design of the delivery plan. Parents said they wanted more practical support, more parenting advice on issues of behaviour management, and information about children's activities. The delivery plan flagged the need for more outreach work and befriending for vulnerable and isolated families and services. The particular needs of asylum-seeker and refugee families were also noted.

The methodology consisted of extensive documentary review of Eight Village Sure Start data and family support models. Parents and carers were consulted via a survey of service users (n=37) and non-service users (n=10), a review of five case study records and six in-depth interviews with users (two with high service users and four to accompany case studies). Nine Sure Start staff and 14 partners were interviewed. The cost-effectiveness of the service was assessed.

The plan

The FSS was to recruit a team of four outreach workers and train volunteers who would work across the area to:

1. work closely with existing services, existing community groups and statutory organisations, such as midwives and health visitors, to provide parents with a network of support

2. act as a befriending service for parents and families, and as a signposting service for Sure Start services and other relevant services within the area

3. encourage parents to identify their own and their children's needs, to seek ways of meeting those needs from the service provided.

In terms of models, the Eight Village Sure Start FSS was originally based on a social services preventative model, but this changed when the SSLP adopted the more holistic Children's Assessment Framework (Department of Health 2000). By placing the child and parent at the centre of a holistic service, which is a core Sure Start value, the model shows that the focus of action or support can cover any issue.

The delivery

An internal review of a sample of 32 closed care plans, covering cases between July 2003 and July 2005, illustrated the type of activity that the service provided (Horton 2005). The sample represents 13 per cent of cases selected from 245 closed files. The analytical framework sought to answer eight core 'who, why, what' type questions:

1. Who refers families to the family support team and where are families posted?

2. Why are families referred to the family support team?

3. Do parents' and carers' own perceptions of their needs differ from reasons for referral?

4. What targets are set within care plans and to what extent are targets met?

5. Are certain types of targets within care plans more likely to be met than others?

6. When families have more needs, are fewer targets likely to be met?

7. Are there any gaps in service provision or training needs?

8. Is paperwork within care plans being filled in appropriately?

Outcomes

The external evaluation showed that the FSS had helped Sure Start to deliver on three out of seven public service agreement (PSA) and service delivery agreement (SDA) targets, mostly health behaviours. User satisfaction was very positive, typically recorded at 97 per cent. The service was responsive, well received and met needs. Over three-quarters (76%) of users said that FSS had made a difference to their life. Parents saw the FSS as the hub for signposting, and over half of onward referrals were to other services (Barton *et al.* 2006). Staff completed 50 home visits for 61 referrals in one year. There were 30 issues in all, but the biggest categories of referrals were play sessions and child development. Targets relating to training and education, play sessions and breastfeeding were most commonly included within care plans (Horton 2005).

Other partners – the statutory services – saw the FSS both as providing extra capacity to undertake work that they considered peripheral to their own core business, and as a follow-on after mainstream provision ended. In effect, it released mainstream capacity. So the FSS met the needs of families, and through collaborative working with statutory agencies added to the total support available. Referrals came mainly from two types of healthcare staff – health visitors and midwives – but parents were slow to self-refer (Barton *et al.* 2006).

One valuable lesson learnt from the internal case study review (Horton 2005) was the need to document activity to produce an evidence-base. The baseline was inadequate for answering external evaluation questions. The lesson was that robust monitoring systems must be set up at the outset of a project like FSS, which has to provide evidence of its impact to justify future funding and mainstreaming. There was scope for improvement in training staff to record casework and for implementing documentation procedures.

We wanted to know the actual level of demand as a proportion of all registered families. The FSS were not able to state the total number of families who had used the service, so it was not possible to show what proportion of Sure Start registered families asked for help. What did families seek support for? The model covers every possible topic, but there was no comprehensive map of topics covered by FSS. What did the service cost? Data on the number of visits were available but took time to be extrapolated from the database. Time was much harder to calculate, given the fluidity of the service and staff working in it, and the work practices of staff unaccustomed to documenting their use of time. Thus, cost-effectiveness was difficult to determine. What changed as a result of FSW input? Cases were closed but outcomes were not recorded.

Thinking through these issues it was clear that the impact of the intervention depended on the complexity of cases. The turnover of families in the catchment area meant that the sampling frame (of registered families) constantly changed. When assessing impact it was noted that some cases needed help which was outside FSS control, such as social services and housing. Some problems were so personal and longstanding that a befriending role was essential, but demand and available resources limit the scope for this.

Discussion

A major part of government policy for children and families is support to enhance parenting skills. In this chapter, we aimed to evaluate the impact of FSS. We have attempted this through reviewing evaluation reports of FSS and through case study, which is not necessarily generalisable. Our evaluation is limited by the problems of having to use weak information systems. Indeed, we conclude that SSLPs face challenges in supplying all the information needed for their external evaluators.

There is no shared theoretical framework for local evaluations, which is a lost opportunity to think through what works where, and in what circumstances. In the early years most local evaluators concentrated on knowledge-building, with some attempts to promote evidence-based policy and practice through case study methods. The change in policy from SSLPs to local authority-led Children's Centres has resulted in a loss of evaluation budget and opportunities, since there is no guarantee that local authorities will be able to fund the same resources.

Our review has been unable to identify any published evaluation reports which discuss or define effectiveness. Few actually measure outputs or attempt to quantify outcomes. An exception to this is the Bentley Children's Centre report (Taylor 2005) on an outreach service, which estimated that over one year the FSS supported 88 families with 119 children. This was thought to be about seven per cent of the total number of families. Most reports document outputs: how many groups, hours, the type of sessions. Few consider mainstreaming or identify examples of innovation or good practice.

Although SSLPs had a dedicated budget for evaluation (between three and five per cent of their funding), this could sometimes be stretched to be more cost-effective, which is not always conducive to a long-term relationship with evaluators. There has sometimes been the compulsion to deliver quick answers. However, programmes grow, change and evolve, so evaluations can only show a snapshot at a particular time. Complex community-based initiatives are hard to evaluate because of their size and the speed with which they change. There can be a multitude of area-based initiatives in SSLP areas, thus demonstrating causality is even more challenging and complicated. Initiatives like Sure Start are trying to address multiple problems in areas of social deprivation which will take decades to change.

Future of FSS

The extent to which local authority-led Children's Centres need to provide FSS should be based on an assessment of the level of provision currently available in the local area. Outreach and home visiting services need to be effective, but we have to know what the measure of effectiveness is. This should be stated at the design stage, linked to formal needs assessment. The aim, objectives and particular goals should be set out in PSA documentation.

Detail about the services offered and levels of take-up is descriptive, secondary data taken from case files. The implicit and explicit assumptions about how this intervention will lead to the desired outcomes need to be transparent and documented as they have the potential to answer the 'what works for whom, why does it work and how does it work?' questions. Service-providers can then apply that learning in other settings. Having these foundations in place is a prerequisite for meaningful evaluation.

Implications for Children's Centres

1. Family Support Services are hard to define and fluid, making comparisons across local programmes problematic, but they are valued by parents, carers and stakeholders.

2. Family Support Services have provided added value and additionality to mainstream services but documenting Family Support activities and outcomes is essential.

3. There are challenges and considerable time lags in demonstrating the outcomes of Family Support Services.

References

Barton, A., Broughton, K., Brooks, L., Jesson, J., Khan, A. and Venus, C. (2006) *Eight Village Sure Start Evaluation of Family Support Service*. Birmingham: M•E•L. Research.

Cordis Bright (2004) *Evaluation 2003/4 Family Support Workers*. Spotlight Report. London: Cordis Bright.

Department of Health (2000) *Framework for the Assessment of Children in Need and their Families*. London: The Stationery Office.

Gardner, R. (2003) *Family Support*. London: Royal Holloway College and Evaluation Department, NSPCC Information Briefings.

Horton, M. (2005) *Review of Family Support Closed Care Plans*. Eight Village Sure Start Local Programme (unpublished).

Outreach Officer (2004) *Evaluation Report: Experience of Ante and Post Natal Visiting in Sandwell*. West Midlands Sandwell Sure Start Citywide (unpublished). www.ness.bbk.ac.uk/documents/findings/848.pdf, accessed on 23 October 2007.

Roberts, T. and Man, S. (2004) *External Evaluation of the Family Support Service (IRIS)*. Bristol: Involving Residents in Solutions.

Taylor, K. (2005) *An Evaluation of the Sure Start Family Support Outreach Service*. Bentley Children's Centre: QA Research (unpublished). www.ness.bbk.ac.uk/documents/findings/1084.pdf, accessed on 23 October 2007.

Weinberger, J. (2003) *A Study of Family Support Work*. Sheffield: Foxhill and Parsons Cross Sure Start.

Part 5

Community Development

Chapter 23

Introduction to Community Development

Paul Leighton

Concerns for modernisation and innovation in public service delivery have led to area based social and healthcare policy initiatives (ABIs) being increasingly commonplace in the UK (Alcock 2004; Hall 2003). Targeted to the most deprived areas, and focused upon regeneration and renewal, programmes such as the New Deal for Communities, the Neighbourhood Renewal Fund and the Education, Employment and Health Action Zones have become integral parts of the UK social policy arena – part of an agenda for creating a more inclusive society. Sure Start is one such ABI – targeted in the most disadvantaged neighbourhoods, working holistically in a multidisciplinary fashion, responsive to local circumstances and sensitive to the local community.

Underpinning this way of working is the belief that the geographic concentration of social problems can create spirals of disadvantage that cannot be tackled by traditional, universal models of social and healthcare service delivery alone. There exists a cumulative 'area' or 'neighbourhood' effect that requires a more targeted form of response. The problem is not unemployment, high crime, poor health, low educational attainment per se but some spatially manifest fusion of these which adds to, and embeds, social, economic and health difficulties (Department of the Environment, Transport and Regions 2000; Forrest and Kearns 1999; Smith 1999; Tunstall and Lupton 2003). ABIs offer 'joined-up solutions' to these interconnected problems, significantly offering a clear and coherent focus for building community capacity, and also for involving local communities in social provision (Alcock 2004, p.93). The justification for area-based investment, therefore, rests not only in the spatial concentration, and complexity, of social and economic problems, but also in the longer-term impact that targeted provision might engender in creating more resilient communities: ABIs '[build] the capacity of the community better to manage the neighbourhood and secure a more prosperous and sustainable longer-term future for the community, after the scheme has been completed' (Department of the Environment, Transport and Regions 2001).

Community is thus significant to Sure Start in two broad ways: as the geographic site for targeted investment, local programmes being planned so that they reflect and 'make sense to the local community' (Department for Education and Skills 2002); but also as a substantive focus for improvement, *strengthening families and communities* being a core Sure Start objective. As Hope and Leighton note in the introduction to Chapter 26, community is both a *goal of service delivery* and also a *mechanism for service delivery*. The coincidence of these two aspects perhaps rests in a broader set of assumptions about the nature of community – that communities are geographically bounded, socially homogeneous and socially and culturally stable. Challenges to this way of thinking are now commonplace (for example, see Castells 1996; Urry 2000), and the chapters presented here offer a more subtle and nuanced interpretation of community in their exploration of local programme experiences. Hope and Leighton draw upon work with a number of SSLPs to explore the changing ways in which community has been conceptualised within the Sure Start agenda, whilst Hamm (Chapter 24), and Bowpitt and Chaudhary (Chapter 25) draw more explicitly upon particular examples of Sure Start service provision to explore issues of race and cultural sensitivity in Sure Start settings.

The chapters by Hamm and by Bowpitt and Chaudhary recognise the varied and differing needs of different parts of the community, and the difficulties that these pose in relation to shaping Sure Start services. Hamm, in her consideration of a multi-ethnic Sure Start area, identifies different patterns of engagement and different patterns of benefit derived by families from different ethnic backgrounds. Asian women were perhaps the most frequent users of Sure Start services in her research, yet they were less active in such things as Sure Start management groups. The resulting *racialised discourse* that she discovered (focused upon perceptions of greater need amongst Asian families) rests in notions of appropriate community participation and subsequently shapes the relationship between the local programme and service users. In a similar vein Bowpitt and Chaudhary focus upon the different, and largely unrecognised, cultural needs of Traveller families. They identify that culturally specific conceptualisations of *family* and *childhood* are largely overlooked in provision that is designed to serve the needs of a local Traveller population. Despite a rhetoric of cultural sensitivity and social inclusiveness, it is mainstream notions of family support which are validated and reinforced in provision, which is unsurprisingly under-utilised by the group for which it is intended.

Both Chapters 24 and 25 identify a gap between policy assumptions about community (uniform and built upon consensus) and the way in which community is played out in local programme settings. Perhaps of more concern is the way in which notions of community have seemingly been applied in an unreflexive fashion, with the differing needs and differing abilities to engage with Sure Start largely overlooked by local programmes in these examples.

The final chapter in Part 5 of this book, by Hope and Leighton (Chapter 26), taps into another assumption that is commonly made about community – that communities are rooted in distinctive geographic spaces with clear and fixed boundaries. In their chapter they recognise that, whilst this assumption might have been more relevant at the outset of Sure Start, when concerns for rebuilding communities and the local management of services were prominent, recent policy developments suggest a more porous and networked understanding of community. This is an understanding of community which is not tied to geographic space but which is linked to participation within broader networks of economic activity, most notably through employment. They suggest that a shift towards a stronger concern for childcare, education and employment advice (as manifest in Children's Centres) can be interpreted in this fashion. They also suggest that the transition from one understanding of community to another has been a site of difficulty and tension for those who deliver and receive Sure Start services.

We have identified elsewhere in this book that Children's Centres are to receive less funding than the former SSLPs, and that their provision is more likely to be prescribed centrally by local government than be led by the concerns of local stakeholders and partnerships. Both these factors suggest not only a more limited role for the community in Children's Centres, they also suggest that community development is less likely to be a core activity. However, the chapters presented here remain pertinent and offer insight that reaches beyond the scope of SSLPs. Specifically they illustrate the complexity of contemporary social and healthcare policy and provision, and the subtlety and sensitivity required to implement such provision in multicultural settings. Both these insights have a relevance to the development and management of Children's Centres.

References

Alcock, P. (2004) 'Participation or pathology.' *Social Policy and Society 3*, 2, 87–96.

Castells, M. (1996) *The Rise of the Network Society*. Oxford: Blackwell.

Department of the Environment, Transport and Regions (2001) *A Review of the Evidence Base for Regeneration Policy and Practice*. London: HMSO.

Department for Education and Skills (2002) *Sure Start, A Guide for Sixth Wave Programmes*. Nottingham: DfES Publications.

Forrest, R. and Kearns, A. (1999) *Joined-up Places? Social Cohesion and Neighbourhood Regeneration*. York: Joseph Rowntree Foundation.

Hall, S. (2003) 'The Third Way revisited: new labour, spatial policy and the national strategy for neighbourhood renewal. *Planning, Practice and Research 18*, 4, 265–277.

Smith, G. (1999) *Area Based Initiatives: The Rationale and Options for Area Targeting*, CASE paper no. 25. www.sticerd.lse.ac.uk/case/publications/casepapers.asp, accessed 9 November 2007.

Tunstall, R. and Lupton, R. (2003) *Is Targeting Deprived Areas An Effective Means to Reach Poor People?* CASE paper no. 70. www.sticerd.lse.ac.uk/case/publications/casepapers.asp, accessed on 9 November 2007.

Urry, J. (2000) *Sociology Beyond Societies: Mobilities for the Twenty-first Century*. London: Routledge.

Chapter 24

Experiences of Parental Involvement in a Multi-ethnic Setting

Tricia Hamm

This chapter examines the Sure Start policy for parental involvement[1] and seeks to understand some aspects of it in one programme area, in particular: who gets involved and what are the outcomes of involvement? Using the concept of human agency to explore parents' experiences, the chapter suggests that parental involvement is shaped by area characteristics, the approach and resources available to the programme, as well as policy messages and requirements. It is suggested that these factors may have unrecognised consequences on the ground – in this case, paying insufficient attention to who participates, and the differential benefits for those who do (and do not) become involved.

The chapter is derived from a broader study which sought to examine how parents engaged with a Sure Start Local Programme. The study was conducted using observational methods and interviews: observation at meetings, groups and events, followed by over 40 in-depth interviews (which included a subset of repeat visits) with white and Asian staff and parents. Fieldwork took place at Sure Start and other community premises and at parents' homes. Interviews were carried out with activist[2] and non-activist parents and used a life-story approach which examined the background and histories of participants, as well as how they viewed and used the Sure Start programme. A narrative analysis approach was adopted which views narratives as 'social products'; as such, they are 'related to the experience that people have of their lives' without being 'transparent carriers of that experience' (Lawler 2002, p.242).

The fieldwork for this study was undertaken during a period of two years from 2003 to 2005 and therefore represents a 'snapshot' of parental involvement at a particular time. Some of the characteristics of involvement, such as the individuals involved, and the Sure Start policy context have subsequently changed. Nonetheless, this snapshot is important in a number of ways: in providing an illustration of tensions between policy assumptions and ground-level experience and in problematising taken-for-granted policy ideas about 'community' and 'community involvement'.

Locating Sure Start in Third Way politics

In this section, I briefly outline theoretical and policy frameworks within which Sure Start can be located and which are used to analyse findings from the study. Since the 1990s, theorists such as Anthony Giddens (1991, 1994) and Ulrich Beck and Elisabeth Beck-Gernsheim (2002) have described an 'individualisation thesis' which states that in our 'de-traditionalised', globalised world of late modernity, identities and individual trajectories are no longer fixed; as 'reflexive agents' we have, instead, an array of lifestyles to choose from and to assemble our own 'life projects'. This 'activation' of *human agency* is incorporated by Giddens into his discussions of Third Way politics and the welfare state (1998). In his thesis on the Third Way, Giddens advocates 'positive welfare' in which the state *enables* active users to access opportunities rather than simply providing benefits and other resources to passive recipients (Williams, Popay and Oakley 1999). The emphasis of a Third Way approach on the development of human capital through the distribution of opportunities, on the responsibilities of individuals alongside their rights, and on the state as enabler defines the Third Way state as a *social investment* state.

In addition, and another key aspect of Giddens' Third Way thesis, the role of politics as defining 'a new relationship between the individual and the community' is described (p.64). Nikolas Rose (2001) identifies a change in the political discourse from social to 'ethical' citizenship; for him, ethopolitics, as he names it, is played out through the terrain of community, with notions of 'responsibility' and 'duty' linked in policy to the improvement of 'degenerated' areas.

Increasing interest in 'community involvement' was evident in Conservative urban policy in the 1990s, but its profile became even more prominent under Labour, influenced by the moralism of Communitarians such as Etzioni (1996) as well as by Third Way ideas. However, in pragmatic terms of policy and practice, the 'slipperiness' of the terms 'community' and 'community involvement' has frequently been noted (Atkinson 1999; Imrie and Waco 2003). Chanan (2003, p.15), for example, highlights the 'unique but somewhat puzzling position of community involvement' which, on the one hand, is a requirement in many public policy arenas, but on the other is often 'vague and ambiguous' and absent from 'outputs, outcomes and budget categories'. He points to the Urban White Paper (Department of the Environment, Transport and Regions 2000) as 'perhaps the nearest thing to a comprehensive framework for government intentions on community involvement' (p.23). Here, he identifies six principles, or purposes of involvement, which he then summarises as a 'triangle of three mutually enhancing objectives': involvement as *governance*; involvement as *social capital*; involvement as *service delivery*. I will be returning to these three policy goals when I examine the outcomes of parental involvement in Brambleton Sure Start.

The Sure Start programme can be located within a Third Way framework. It is an example of 'social investment' policy, future-focused with the 'investment' being in the human capital of parents and children (Lister 2003). Sure Start guidance documents repeatedly describe parents as 'aspirational', and as active agents wanting to make the 'right' decisions for their children by taking advantage of opportunities for training and paid work and by improving their parenting.

Parental involvement, while entirely voluntary in Sure Start, also fits within Third Way understandings of community as a vehicle of social cohesion and inclusion (Fremeaux 2005). Norman Glass, the 'architect of Sure Start', highlights parental involvement as a unique strength of the Sure Start vision.

> This programme would be 'owned' by local parents, local communities and those who worked in the programme. Because those who benefited would be able to shape it to do what they wanted, rather than it being to, or for, them. (The Guardian, 5 January 2005)

In the early days of Sure Start there was immense optimism about the potential of parental involvement, especially given that Sure Start had been announced as a ten-year programme. Prospective Sure Start programmes were required to undertake intensive community consultation, and in Brambleton's delivery plan, it was stated that parents were to be kept 'at the heart of the programme, shaping the services that are delivered'.

However, community involvement in Sure Start was arguably characterised by various tensions – the grand claims made about parent ownership contrasting with a weak practical application in terms of implementation, and accountability being a key example. Within policy documents themselves, parental involvement was highlighted as essential, but treated as a technical task, rather than being seen as in any way problematic or complex. In Brambleton many professionals discussed their concerns about a *downgrading* of parental involvement, particularly with the introduction of Children's Centres and their incorporation into local authorities. The perceived downgrading of parental involvement during this period can also be seen in guidance documents themselves. In Sure Start objectives, for example, there is arguably a shift in tone from an emphasis on *governance* (in Chanan's terms) to *social capital* in the relevant objective ('Strengthening Families and Communities'), and a parallel shift in the changes to the 'key principles'.[3,4]

The case study: Brambleton as a 'racialised' area

Brambleton is one of the smallest Sure Start areas in England. It is geographically isolated, located on the edge of a northern city with no bordering residential areas. Census data (2001) indicate that there were two major ethnic groupings within the area, with white residents the largest group (52%), and those of British Asian ethnicity the second largest (41%). Within the Asian group, those identifying as Asian–Pakistani formed a large majority (91%). The age profile of the Asian–Pakistani group was markedly younger than that of white residents; however, there were still sizeable numbers of children aged 0–4 identified as white (35% of this age group, that is, 115 children, compared with 57% of Asian–Pakistani children, 192 children). As the study focused on white and Pakistani-origin mothers, in the remainder of the chapter, the latter will be referred to as 'Asian'.

Monitoring data and 2001 Census data suggested in 2004 that just over a half of Asian families were registered with Brambleton Sure Start (BSS) whereas the comparable proportion for the white population was under one-fifth. In a year spent observing Sure Start groups and meetings, I saw very few white women service users – perhaps a handful – other than those who were 'activists'. However, during the fieldwork period, out of five mothers who were active, that is, regular members of the Parent's Group, only one was Asian. In addition, across the whole sample the white women demonstrated different characteristics to those of the Asian women. For example, three had degrees, where none of the Asian women had, and all of the white women had moved into the area relatively recently, whereas the large majority of the Asian women had lived in Brambleton since childhood, most having extended family nearby.

A central theme in the study is the construction of Brambleton as a 'racialised' space by professionals and residents (Smith 1989). Interviews with professionals concerning the rationale and continuing need for Sure Start provision defined the area as 'Asian'; staff saw many of the local Asian women as isolated, lacking in autonomy, sometimes as 'victims' of patriarchal families. This led to an assumption that a particular need for Sure Start services lay with these women, with little recognition at that point given to characteristics and needs of other population groups in Brambleton.[5]

Brambleton was also seen as historically neglected by services. Early interviews describe how Asian women, frustrated by the lack of childcare and activities for mothers, came together with professionals to develop the Brambleton Childcare Project (BCP), subsequently the lead body for Sure Start. This story of BCP, revealed largely through interviews with staff who were asked about the origins of Sure Start in Brambleton, tells of the triumph of community involvement, with Asian women taking on a heroic role in the struggle for better services. While Asian women continue to be highly involved in BCP Management Committee, the picture at Sure Start is very different.

Parent involvement in Brambleton Sure Start

In Brambleton, there were two main avenues for parental involvement. The first of these, the Parent's Group, had various roles: functioning as a social and discussion forum, initiating new Sure Start groups, and developing a range of activities to draw in a wider section of the local population. The Management Board was the regular decision-making multi-agency meeting which included a slot for feedback from the Parent's Group. Parent attendance was patchy at both of these groups, despite ongoing attempts to improve participation. At Management Board meetings there would, on occasion, be no representation at all, although during the later stages of the fieldwork a parent would chair this meeting whilst attendance by other parents remained very low. For a short time three of the white activist parents became active volunteers in different areas of the programme.

In the remainder of the chapter, I explore the particular character of parental involvement in Brambleton. I will argue that a lack of coherence and accountability at policy level, the relatively small resources that the programme could offer this issue, and the 'racialised' understanding of the area resulted in a narrow approach to involvement, which could not fundamentally recognise or address the differential capacity to become involved, and the resulting varying impact for different groups.

Motivation and outcomes

The notion of involvement as 'the right thing to do', or as an expression of 'ethical citizenship', featured highly in the accounts of those who were actively involved. These accounts stress the 'right' and 'duty' to 'have a say', and reflect the policy goals that Chanan (2003) has referred to, particularly those of governance and service delivery. Not surprisingly, involvement for these white parent activists is also described as fulfilling, enjoyable and as functioning as a counter to the 'mundane' routine of childrearing.

> I want to influence what happens in my community, because I want to make it better, and if I can make it better then I'll be doing something good for my kids and I'll be doing something good for all the other children. (Nicola)

> We're living in this area, we have a right to decide what can happen in the area, what we want to see, so why not? The party, that was my idea, and it gives you a sense of "that was down to us". It just gives you a sense of authority. And we have as much an involvement in Brambleton as the people that work here. (Kerry)

> And I think you get out of it the fact that, you know, you've got some like-minded parents that turn up. And I mean, it's good fun as well. (Emma)

The study indicates that parental involvement resulted in some discernible effects on provision, in the form of parent organisation of one-off events and short-term groups. However, despite rhetorical commitment to a governance approach in which parents were key partners, there was no fundamental input into the direction of the programme by parents.[6] In practical terms, there was greatest commitment from staff, and largest impacts for parents, in terms of individual capacity-building.

> I never thought I'd go to something as official as the Board Meeting in my life. Never have voiced my opinion like that, as much as I'm quite a mouthy person. But it's taught me a lot more about people... I don't think I'd have been sitting here, say, three years ago, I never would have walked into a room, with people who – gobbledy-gooked as such. (Kerry)

Theorists have identified three types of social capital: *bonding capital*, which represents strong social ties between like individuals such as family or an ethnic grouping; *bridging capital*, which concerns weaker ties that cut across social groups; and *linking capital* which represents vertical connections, such as relationships between social classes, and between the powerful and less powerful (described in Kearns 2004). The study suggests that parent activists in this period, particularly those who became volunteers, gained access to the most powerful form of social capital, *linking capital*, through this process. Through activities initiated at the Parent's Group, attending the Management Board and in their volunteer roles, these women received intensive input and experience which gave them specific skills, support and contacts. Here, volunteering is described by Helen as orientated explicitly towards developing work skills.

> It's very much about developing capacity, they get a chance to see people at work, they see the work environment and know how that feels, they get to know some of the systems, meetings. We expect a certain kind of professional behaviour and that's been achieved in many ways. (Helen)

Parents who had become volunteers also identified that the experience had precipitated their interest in looking for paid work and, moreover, employment in a Sure Start-related field.

> Before I started volunteering there was no way I would have thought about applying for a job. (Nicola)

> Has it changed the way you look at future work? (Researcher)

> Definitely, definitely. I mean now, if I don't get [the job that I've applied for at Sure Start], I will definitely be looking for other work in similar areas. (Nicola)

> If there was a position here, in two months' time, then of course I'll go for it. I've got the experience now, this has built my confidence up. (Kerry)

'Involvement' and 'non-involvement' as a reflection of a racialised dynamic

Parents who used Sure Start services, but were not activists, gave a variety of reasons for this. But narratives around *non-involvement* often reflected racialised stories about the Asian women in the area and the difficulties that they experienced in using services more generally.[7]

A theme within the wider study looks at how the notion of 'constrained agency' can be applied particularly to some of the Asian women in the sample.[8] This contests the individualisation thesis advocated by Giddens and Beck, suggesting in particular that the premise of 'de-traditionalisation', upon which this thesis rests, has been overstated – an observation made by others who have explored agency in cultural and religious groups (Wray 2004; Yip 2004). Below, Helen roots many of these women firmly in family and community obligations; their *agency*, their *capacity to act*, is, in her view, significantly delimited by what they have to do for others.

> Culturally, many women, especially Asian women, have never really had much for themselves, and along comes Sure Start, offering this, offering that, in return we'd like to have thought, for parental involvement. But in fact these women have very little left, they've got nothing else to give. What they need is time for themselves, in order to kind of re-charge their batteries and that may well take three years. For many, you can just see that can't feature in their lives, because there's that one tiny bit of time for themselves, and they've the kids in the crèche, and they've got an hour. That hour means that they can stay sane, and they can't come to a group where they might have – some other local parents – mouthing off about this, that and the other. (Helen)

Some aspects of this narrative were described by other participants, including a small number of the Asian women interviewed, who emphasised language barriers and the weight of household and family obligations.

> I don't know if it's our cooking that takes a long time or what it is. It might be that they want to come but they don't know English, you know – they want to put their voice across but they won't know if there's anyone to put their voice to. Or they've never been and they don't know how to go. (Nazia)

Helen's point earlier that women were actively choosing to protect their time by not becoming involved is given another perspective by accounts about involvement in the Brambleton Childcare Project (see earlier). Below, Shamim identifies that she became involved with BCP because, with children now at school, she at last had the time to do something for herself.

> I think the majority of the women who were round at my time, they didn't have kids at home, right, they'd their housework but they still had a lot of time. Once my kids went to school I was looking for somewhere where I could socialise, just go out and have a nice chat, you know, do swimming. I wasn't even thinking about – going back into work or going and doing training. I just wanted some time out to myself, that was all I was looking for. (Shamim)

This is reflected also in discussion with a BCP worker who tries to identify why Asian women had been drawn to involvement in her organisation rather than in Sure Start.

> It is a pull that they see it as childcare, where they can leave their children, and then go and do something else, whether it's training or being a volunteer, being part of the Management Committee, being involved in meetings while your child is – doing their own thing. At Sure Start, I think it's perceived to be different, most of their meetings will offer childcare but I think it's the things that might come from that, it's all *with* your children. (Karen)

While these stories generally stressed factors which *constrained* Sure Start involvement, some white participants tapped into a very different narrative which was about Asian women *making use of services but giving nothing back*. This is another aspect of the racialised dynamics which includes how different groups constructed each other in this area. Lisa's comments reflect others by white staff who appear to wish to show empathy, but also suggest a tentativeness and uncertainty about how 'other' lives are lived.

> I supported a parent with her job application, and another parent I've been taking training, but these are actually white parents. I can only sort of say this 'cause I spoke to colleagues who are Asian that live in the community. They've said, 'When it's just something like a meeting, they're not going to want to get involved'. If it's something nice, you know, where you can take the children to get a break, or it's something they're getting out of it [then they'll do it]. (Lisa)

Some white parents were harsher in their analysis. For example, Kerry's description of the women (as selfish, 'moaning to their husbands') contrasts significantly with that of some of the staff who spoke of Asian women in very different terms – as selfless, uncomplaining, passive.

> People moan and complain about what doesn't happen in Brambleton. Well we have the opportunity to come and put things forward, but people don't come. They're willing to take up the trips, the courses, everything, but they're not willing to give any input back. They're probably moaning to their husbands 'I wish there was this' or 'I wish there was that' or 'I didn't like the way this trip was run'. (Kerry)

> So why don't people get involved? (Researcher)

> Can't be bothered? Quite happy maybe to let other people do it? We've gone to every single meeting, we think it's our duty to come. (Kerry)

Conclusions

A focus here on human agency suggests that policy assumptions about an undifferentiated capacity to engage with interventions (in this case the Sure Start programme) are simplistic, may fail to address difficulties of engagement, or recognise the differential impacts that policies may have on different groups. These findings, about agency as nuanced and mediated by social factors, are supported by the work of commentators such as Hoggett whose 2001 model challenges current policy notions that the self must always be active and reflexive (Hoggett 2001), and by those (e.g. Mason 2004) who have explored agency as gendered and 'relational', not intrinsic to the individual, but often highly constrained by the demands of others.

A second related component of Third Way politics – a vision of 'community' as consensual, as essentially beyond politics and as a vehicle for social cohesion – is also challenged by these findings. Explorations of agency and *perceptions* of the agency of others illuminated how groups constructed and interacted with each other in Brambleton. In other parts of the study, white and Asian mothers expressed positive feelings about living in a multi-ethnic area. However, white activist parents occasionally expressed ignorance and negativity about their Asian counterparts. The dominance of these relatively confident and empowered white women in parental involvement structures may itself have been one of the contributory factors in the unwillingness of other parents to become involved.

On a practical level, this study suggests that the treatment of parental involvement in an inconsistent and sometimes contradictory way at the level of policy impacted upon what could be done locally. In policy documents parental involvement is extolled, but not resourced or subject to targets, and is treated essentially as a technical task. In Brambleton, there was concern about the lack of active parents, but there was not any overarching strategic attempt to understand or address this. Moreover, because of the 'racialisation' of Brambleton, with Asian women seen often as 'victims' and in greatest need of Sure Start services, at this point strategies to support them to become more actively involved were not explored.

The lack of resources and targets for parental involvement also had large implications for the focus of this work. While there was in Brambleton Sure Start a sincere commitment to a governance approach in the form of partnership with parents, there were difficulties in translating this into reality. In practice, much of the work in this area focused, very successfully, on developing the individual capacity of involved parents. During this period, therefore, white women activists were the major beneficiaries of this intensive input. In fact, these women are all now in paid employment: two in local organisations with links to BSS and two now resident outside of the area. To return to the policy goals that Chanan identified (2003), described earlier in this chapter, a final and not unusual irony is revealed: the greater emphasis on *social capital*, rather than governance or service delivery, meant that this very social capital, accrued through a group of white parents with less investment in the area, was more likely to leave, rather than remain in Brambleton and contribute to its regeneration.

Implications for Children's Centres

- Policy assumptions about an undifferentiated capacity to engage with social and healthcare interventions are simplistic and fail to address the difficulties that parts of the community experience in engaging with them or, similarly, to recognise the differential impacts that policies may have on different groups.

- Notions that 'community' is consensual and beyond politics (i.e. a natural vehicle for social cohesion) are also simplistic, and fail to recognise the way in which different social and ethnic groups construct and interact with each other.

- Inconsistencies in the treatment of parental involvement at a policy level (i.e. extolled but not resourced) have a negative impact upon what might be achieved locally.

Acknowledgements

The author would like to thank Barbara Rimmington for her thoughts and comments on the chapter and for her valuable ongoing contribution to the study.

Notes

1   In this chapter parental involvement is treated as a form of community involvement; in the policy literature, the term 'parental involvement' is usually found in literature on schools and education.

2   The term 'activist' is used to describe those who were involved in parent involvement forums or activities.

3   In 2001, the subheading to the objective was 'In particular, *by involving families in building the community's capacity to sustain the programme and thereby create pathways out of poverty'*. By 2003, this had changed to 'By encouraging all providers of children's services to take a wider view of their role in the community and, in particular in disadvantaged areas, *by involving families in building capacity in the community and creating pathways out of poverty'* (my emphasis).

4   The early emphasis in two of six 'key principles' on involvement which built on the 'existing strengths' of family members and carers, and on participation of 'all local families in the design and working of the programme', was replaced in 2003 by a less active conceptualisation, arguably in the language of consumerism: services were to be 'customer driven'; there should be 'consultation and day-to-day listening to parents'.

5   Given the relatively large number of white and other young children in the area, this is a striking finding and is further addressed in the wider study.

6   It was noted that some major decisions, for example, those concerning finance, were often taken by BSS staff *away* from Board Meetings. A governance approach was more evident in another local programme (in which a small amount of comparative work was conducted). For example, at this second programme, in order to be quorate, at least four parents had to be present, parent activists attended a facilitated preparatory group before each Board meeting, and *all* significant decisions were taken at Board Meetings.

7   It is important to note here a methodological point about the difficulties in talking about non-involvement with those who were not active (as if involvement were the *acceptable* norm).

8   It is important to emphasise that this situation is dynamic, that roles, possibilities, trajectories for this group are in flux. Several women who were interviewed demonstrated this, in their descriptions of how they both *acquiesced in* and *contested* expectations of them.

References

Atkinson, R. (1999) 'Discourses of partnership and empowerment in contemporary British urban regeneration.' *Urban Studies 36*, 1, 59–72.

Beck, U. and Beck-Gernsheim, E. (2002) *Individualisation.* London: Sage.

Chanan, G. (2003) *Searching for Solid Foundations, Community Involvement and Urban Policy.* London: Office of the Deputy Prime Minister.

Department of the Environment, Transport and Regions (2000) *Our Towns and Cities: the Future. Delivering an Urban Renaissance.* London: Office of the Deputy Prime Minister.

Etzioni, A. (1996) *The New Golden Rule: Community and Morality in a Democratic Society.* New York, NY: Basic Books.

Fremeaux, I. (2005) 'New Labour's appropriation of the concept of community: a critique.' *Community Development Journal 40*, 3, 265–274.

Giddens, A. (1991) *Modernity and Self-Identity: Self and Society in the Late Modern Age.* Cambridge: Polity Press.

Giddens, A. (1994) 'Living in a Post-Traditional Society.' In U. Beck, A. Giddens and S. Lash (eds) *Reflexive Modernization, Politics, Tradition and Aesthetics in the Modern Social Order.* Cambridge: Polity Press.

Giddens, A. (1998) *The Third Way – The Renewal of Social Democracy.* Cambridge: Polity Press.

Glass, N. (2005) 'Surely some mistake.' *Society Guardian*, 5 January.

Hoggett, P. (2001) 'Agency, rationality and social policy.' *Journal of Social Policy 30*, 1, 37–56.

Imrie, R. and Waco, M. (2003) 'Community and the changing nature of urban policy.' In R. Imrie and M. Raco (eds) *Urban Renaissance? New Labour, Community and Urban Policy.* Bristol: Policy Press.

Kearns, A. (2004) *Social Capital, Regeneration and Urban Policy.* CNR Paper 15. www.bristol.ac.uk/sps/cnrpaperspdf/cnr15pap.pdf, accessed on 23 August 2007.

Lawler, S. (2002) 'Narrative in Social Research.' In T. May (ed) *Qualitative Research in Action.* London: Sage.

Lister, R. (2003) 'Investing in the citizen-workers of the future: transformations in citizenship and the state under New Labour.' *Social Policy and Administration 37*, 5, 427–443.

Mason, J. (2004) 'Personal narratives, relational selves: residential histories in the living and the telling.' *Sociological Review 52*, 2, 162–179.

Office for National Statistics (2002) *Census.* Titchfield: Crown Copyright.

Rose, N. (2001) 'Community, citizenship and the Third Way.' In D. Meredyth and J. Minson (eds) *Citizenship and Cultural Policy.* London: Sage.

Smith, S. (1989) *The Politics of 'Race' and Residence.* London: Polity Press.

Williams, F., Popay, J. and Oakley, A. (1999) 'Changing Paradigms of Welfare.' In F. Williams, J. Popay and A. Oakley (eds) *Welfare Research, A Critical Review.* London: UCL Press.

Wray, S. (2004) 'What constitutes agency and empowerment for women in later life?' *Sociological Review 52*, 1, 22–38.

Yip, A. (2004) 'Negotiating space with family and kin in identity construction: the narratives of British non-heterosexual Muslims.' *Sociological Review 52*, 3, 337–350.

Chapter 25

Inclusion and Diversity: Issues for Travellers

Graham Bowpitt and Sarah Chaudhary

This chapter provides an account of an evaluation of a nursery scheme operating exclusively for Gypsy families. The service involved the funding of nursery places by a local Sure Start programme based in a deprived ward with substantial social housing on the edge of a Midlands city. Within its boundaries was a Traveller site populated by Gypsies of Irish heritage (referred to interchangeably throughout the text as 'Gypsies' or 'Travellers'). The scheme was targeted at the Gypsy families as part of Sure Start's hard-to-reach strategy, the aim of which was the inclusion and engagement of minority populations under Sure Start auspices. The evaluation was originally intended to explore user satisfaction. However, consideration of the findings in the light of the literature on Gypsy culture and the multiculturalist and social inclusion agendas of Sure Start posed wider questions about the relationship between a highly conservative, minority culture and the state provision of Early Years welfare services.

This chapter addresses the debate surrounding multiculturalism and how it relates to social inclusion. This debate has become a key policy concern with the establishment of the Commission for Integration and Cohesion. This government advisory body is charged not only with considering the potential benefits of the increasing levels of diversity within communities but also with addressing the tensions and difficulties that increased diversity can cause. At its inauguration, Ruth Kelly, the then Secretary of State for Communities and Local Government, questioned whether a commitment to multiculturalism encourages the separateness that undermines social cohesion (Kelly 2006). Several related questions follow. What does a multiculturalist approach to social policy amount to in practice? Can multicultural services respect and promote diverse cultures at the same time as promoting inclusion within a specific, value-based policy agenda, or will minority cultural identities always be lost to a process of cultural assimilation? Whose culture is being advocated through Sure Start, and are its values compatible with the cultures it claims to support?

Little has been written about Gypsies that specifically focuses on pre-school services. OFSTED noted the low participation rate of Traveller children and the traditional reluctance of families to place young children in formal educational settings (OFSTED 1996, p.24). More recent research has highlighted the serious educational disadvantages that follow from this non-engagement with the education system, with Gypsy and Traveller children showing the poorest achievement of any ethnic minority groups in all Key Stages (Department for Education and Skills 2005). Meanwhile, the National Evaluation of the Children's Fund has provided evidence of the inaccessibility of children's leisure services to children from these minority groups (Mason *et al.* 2006).

The impact of environmental factors on the socialisation of very young children is well known (Sure Start Unit 2005), while child rearing in the early years is an important medium for expressing cultural assumptions and ensuring cultural continuity (Dwivedi 2002, p.47). As Sure Start is rolled out into a national network of Children's Centres, it is hoped that the case study described in this chapter will illuminate the barriers that prevent conservative minority cultures from engaging with Early Years services (Home Office 2005, p.23) and challenge some of the simplistic and unproblematic ways in which concepts of multiculturalism and inclusiveness have been applied to policy and practice.

The evaluation of the nursery scheme comprised five semistructured interviews with service providers at management and operational levels who were involved with the project either through Sure Start, the nursery itself or Traveller outreach services at the County Council. A series of informal conversations was also held with six local Gypsy parents, four of whose children had used the service. These conversations took place in a variety of unusual settings, as it is common practice for Gypsies to maintain a position of control through ensuring that meetings are held on their terms (Levinson and Sparks 2003, p.588). Only after numerous informal conversations had been held were more formal meetings possible, where concurrent notes could be taken. Similarly, the topics covered reflected the Gypsies' apparent need to maintain control: much of the time was spent discussing very specific complaints about the Traveller services and Sure Start, for example delays in the supply of free home safety equipment, or unfairness in the uneven allocation of benefits within the Traveller community. These complaints were fed back informally to the relevant service providers as well as written up in the formal evaluation report. However, within these conversations, broader issues relating to culture, such as religion, education, the responsibility for childcare, conceptions of the family and the status and role of children, were discussed.

The Nursery Project: background and controversies

The initial evaluation question about the effectiveness of the nursery scheme did not take long to answer. Take-up of places proved to be extremely low, with many unfilled for large parts of the year. During the six-month period of investigation, a maximum of three children were in attendance, despite capacity for up for ten. This is in contrast to the situation of non-Traveller families who had to spend some months on a waiting list before being able to take up a nursery place. Our investigation was therefore mainly concerned with finding out the reasons for this low take-up.

At a superficial level, there were likely to be difficulties arising from the way the scheme was set up and managed. The decision to fund the project was taken without any discussion with representatives of the Traveller community or relevant agencies regarding the complex ways in which that community might be affected. Moreover, there was no consideration of the appropriateness of the County Council's policy of using only mainstream, rather than on-site, service provision, despite extensive literature expressing disquiet about this practice (Adams *et al.* 1975, p.109; O'Hanlon and Holmes 2004, p.18; Worrall 1979, pp.54–90). The views of some of the local Gypsy parents that, for instance, 'It's better if all the [Traveller] children are schooled together...we're not used to giving up the children', were similarly not taken into account.

A further concern was that the nursery places were paid for a year in advance, despite ignorance of likely take-up. Moreover, some Sure Start staff felt the scheme discriminated against non-Gypsy families who were thus denied childcare places due to lack of capacity, whilst the Travellers' places remained largely unfilled. This was despite comparable problems of deprivation and low literacy amongst some of the settled community in this area. In other words, no case for positive discrimination could be made in terms of greater need. It is somewhat paradoxical that a service supposedly grounded so firmly in the principle of *inclusiveness* should be offered *exclusively* to one specific community.

Two communities, two cultures

According to the accounts given by local service providers, the aim of the nursery project was to provide a 'culturally relevant, vibrant and holistic [nursery] service for children aged between two and five years'. However, the non take-up of nursery places is unsurprising when we recognise that, far from promoting cultural inclusiveness, Sure Start has its own moral and cultural assumptions that are at odds with those of this Traveller community, and, we would argue, those of other minorities that the Sure Start and New Labour projects have sought to embrace. Table 25.1 identifies the key points of distinction between the cultures of Sure Start and the Irish Gypsies.

Table 25.1 Sure Start and Gypsy childcare values

Cultural Practice	Sure Start	Gypsy Culture
Breastfeeding	Heavily promoted	Strongly discouraged
Pregnancy	Celebrated	Disguised where possible
Gender roles	Largely undifferentiated	Pronounced
Religion	Secular pluralist stance	Christian faith of paramount importance
Social inclusion	Promoted as a core value	Historic dissociation from 'Gorgio' culture
Fighting	Strictly proscribed	Key to masculinity
Literacy	Important goal	Indifference beyond basic level
Toys and play	Fundamental to child development	Little use of toys for play or learning
Childcare	Institutionalised childcare central to Sure Start	Devolved to female members of family
Family values	Egalitarian, pluralist	Patriarchal, traditional

Family and childcare

Commentators confirm the absolute centrality of traditional family values as the most important aspect of Gypsies' self-identity (Fisher 2004, pp.4–12; Greenfields 2006; McCarthy 1994, pp.121–130), and so it was always likely that service use would be mainly limited to families where these values were at risk (Acton 1974, pp.35–36). The Travellers we spoke to confirmed that the family and Christianity were the most important factors that held their society together and distinguished it from the mainstream culture.

However, service providers seemed oblivious to the possibility that such a traditional value system might be relevant to the take-up of nursery services, and that the value system in which their own agencies and services are grounded may be incompatible with this fundamental aspect of Gypsy culture. The response of service providers to the low take-up rates was simply to 'demand we get more children in' rather than to acknowledge that the lack of success of the service might represent an assertion of cultural autonomy by the Traveller families. There appeared to be a firm belief that institutionalised childcare must be in everyone's interest. In this, Sure Start was reproducing the long-held cultural presumptions of liberal service providers regarding the universal desirability of the services being proffered (Acton 1974, p.273).

The status of children within the family unit is seen as a distinguishing feature of the Gypsy family. Judith Okely (1983, pp.159–161) describes how:

> children are highly valued by all members of the group... They are never voluntarily handed over to Gorgios [a perjorative term for settled people]. Disapproval was directed towards people who voluntarily left their children to strangers, the practice being regarded as an attribute of Gorgios not Gypsies.

Other commentators agree (Adams *et al.* 1975, pp.55–91; Greenfields 2006, p.43), pointing out that the most important role of the family is children's socialisation, especially with regard to religious, moral or health practices. One of the clearest distinctions between Gypsies and settled people is that Gypsies maintain the means of socialisation within the family, whereas settled people have transferred this role to institutions. This view was supported by the Travellers in our study, one of whom insisted, 'Why would I be giving them out to strangers... I don't want some stranger bringing up my children giving them ideas'.

Extension of the role of public sector organisations in the socialisation of children will therefore undermine the distinctiveness of Gypsy culture, with the accompanying risks of assimilation and cultural amalgamation. Distinct and separate services can only be justified for a group if it can claim to have a discrete culture (Hawes and Perez 1996, p.37; Worral 1979, p.12). As the fundamental distinctions between lifestyles are whittled away through participation in mainstream services, such justifications will diminish. The result will be services that are essentially the same in terms of fundamental values, but which pay lip service to diversity in a superficial, fetishist way, for example through the possession of 'ethnic' toys or pictures, what Hawes and Perez (1996, p.84) refer to as a 'reservation' or 'gift industry' view of Gypsy culture.

The Gypsies' moral conception of the family is also at odds with Sure Start's moral pluralism that treats all contemporary family forms, such as lone parenthood or cohabitation, as morally equivalent, in contrast to the primacy of marriage advocated by Gypsies (Greenfields 2006, pp.33–36). The Traveller parents in this research perceived this moral disparity in even starker terms with one mother castigating agencies such as Sure Start for being mainly concerned with 'single mothers...drug addicts and drinkers...it's them that gets all the help'. This was one Gypsy perception of the injustices of Sure Start's targeting the neediest, for instance, through its 'hard-to-reach' strategies. By seeking to incorporate Gypsies into its Early Years programme, Sure Start is exposing them to a moral system very different from the one that has traditionally underpinned their culture.

However, a number of Traveller families did choose to attend the nursery. Did this imply a dilution of traditional family values? More likely it reflects a degree of cultural heterogeneity, with community members displaying different levels of internalisation of group norms and reflecting the influence of the dominant culture to varying degrees. This can be extremely problematic within some minority communities, whose highly conservative outlook on life can result in anything from minor disapproval to systematic avoidance of those who deviate from its accepted mores (Greenfields 2006, p.39). Services such as the nursery scheme could therefore be seen as a means by which deviants excluded from the support networks of the minority community can escape the impact of its sanctions. Although this might be justified in terms of reaching out towards excluded families, it does not sit easily with the service's multiculturalist claims. Services that provide a refuge to those deviating from community norms are endorsing the deviant's choice and undermining community sanctions and the values that underpin them. Such services cannot therefore be said to be upholding or supporting the minority culture.

Childhood and play

Further cultural contradictions arise from the differences between Travellers' and mainstream conceptions of the position and role of children in society. The Gypsy understanding of childhood is fundamentally different from that of mainstream society (Greenfields 2006; Okely 1983, pp.160–183). Gypsy children have always developed and learned within the adult world of work and family. 'Play' for them is based on those things that will form a part of their lives as functioning members of the adult economy, such as working on car engines, rag sorting and the raising of livestock. By contrast, for Sure Start, toys and play are fundamental to children's development and learning. Services such as Baby's First Play Pack, Language through Toys and Play and the posts of specific Play Workers all exemplify this.

The local Sure Start programme was committed to 'promoting the importance of play [and] specifically addressing [the Travellers'] lack of smaller play resources'. Consequently, part of the nursery scheme's remit was to broaden the experiences of Traveller children. The implication from Traveller service literature and the Children's Fund research (Mason *et al.* 2006, p.35) is that Traveller children are deprived, experientially as well as materially. Yet the breadth of experience that comes from growing up in a Gypsy community is not recognised.

This raises further questions regarding the respect for Gypsies' autonomy and ability to make choices and decisions for themselves, according to their own criteria of worth. The importance of play is presented in the Sure Start literature as a universally accepted norm, not something relative to the nature, aims and aspirations of different cultures at different times and places. But on what grounds is the claim based that play is important within the Gypsy way of life, society and economy? By emphasising cultural artefacts, such as toys, that have no value to Travellers' ways of life and failing to attach importance to those things that do, such as their traditional methods of learning, agencies such as Sure Start are likely to undermine Gypsies' ability to maintain their own independent economy and culture.

When challenged with this point, one outreach worker appealed once again to the argument from cultural deprivation. 'You can't deny Traveller children the things other children have got. These are some of the most deprived people in [this area]; they can't afford all the toys and other equipment that we take for granted'. This well-meaning concern masks an ignorance of this aspect of the culture of Gypsies that denies them the autonomy to shape the lives of their own children. It implies that Gypsies are mere victims of poverty, rather than positively asserting a view of childhood as a facet of a distinct culture, demanding deliberate actions to sustain Travellers' identity as an autonomous community.

This is not to say that all the families we spoke to maintain the Gypsy view of childhood unequivocally. Only a few feared the nursery's potential to undermine their culture. For instance, one mother lamented, 'They're pure spoiled a lot of the children now... All this nursery and school gets to them. They treat them too babyish so they think they can do as they want'.

Most respondents did not see it as problematic that children should be together with those of a similar age, in an environment specifically created for children. Whether this view was the result of exposure to children's services or other factors is unclear. Certainly the change was recent, as respondents noted that it was 'not at all like when we were young. We were always with, you know, older sisters and cousins, not all together playing as children... You were always on the site or on the road'. Participation in designated children's services therefore appears to be an aspect of the mainstream culture that some Traveller families prefer to their own and to which they are happy to demur. We were unable to discern the prevalence of this view in the Traveller community generally, but the threat that it represents to Gypsy cultural distinctiveness is clear.

However, it was attitudes to toys that revealed the sharpest conflict of values. It was partly that respondents felt that Sure Start's emphasis was encouraging children to be materialistic through 'spoiling them with toys'. This was, apart from anything else, undesirable for practical reasons in undermining the tradition of being prepared to set off at any time, without the need for extensive preparations. But it was Sure Start's use of 'culturally reflective' toys that proved particularly problematic. Some families saw this as downright insulting by insinuating that Gypsies need to learn about their own culture from service providers who had no real understanding of it. Pictures of horses and wagons were seen as representing a mythologised past that did not reflect the Travellers' lived experiences. One mother asserted:

> It's just about being a Gypsy to them... I never been in a wagon in my life; we have trailers and caravans... What do they know about Travelling? I want my children to learn reading and writing... If they want to learn about being a Traveller, can't I take them to their grandma?

The real irony is that, to be genuinely culturally reflective, Gypsy children would not be given toys at all.

Conclusion

This case study of a Sure Start scheme for providing nursery places for the exclusive use of Traveller families reveals what happens when superficially attractive political mantras about multiculturalism and inclusiveness are applied unreflectively in practice. Service providers were dissatisfied with the low take-up of places on this project and yet this did not lead to a questioning of its appropriateness or any acknowledgement of the ways in which Sure Start's own value system might be incompatible with that of the Gypsy community. The scheme was at odds with virtually all the cultural practices and values that are widely regarded as being central to Gypsy culture and which distinguish it from mainstream society, the most important of these being the respective roles of families and institutions in the raising of young children. By encroaching upon a family structure so central to the traditional Gypsy way of life, Sure Start can be seen as continuing decades of a welfare policy that has sought to undermine that way of life and assimilate the Gypsies into the dominant culture.

The design of the Sure Start nursery scheme, for which recognition of a distinct world of childhood expressed through toys and play was fundamental, was at odds with the Gypsy practice of raising children in the context of adult experience. Moreover, the unique experiences of Gypsy children were devalued or dismissed by those involved in the scheme, while Gypsy culture was trivialised by the inappropriate use of 'culturally reflective' toys. Despite claiming to provide a 'culturally appropriate' service, the scheme actually offered a prescriptive, mainstream model rooted in Sure Start values. In the light of the susceptibility of young children to external influences, it would be difficult to claim that this scheme would have anything other than assimilationist effects. Service providers stated that a mainstream model was necessary in order to fulfil the aims of a social inclusion agenda. That so few families chose to be included is perhaps indicative of the limits to this agenda and its greater desirability amongst service providers and policy makers than those whom it is intended to include.

The implications of this study for Children's Centres might appear to be somewhat bleak. The New Labour government appears increasingly anxious about the position of Gypsy children in the education performance tables and more widely about the security implications of preserving minority cultures that thrive on their 'separateness'. This will increase the pressure for Gypsy children to succeed in mainstream education. Against this view, this study points to the need for on-site provision for Gypsy and Traveller communities, at least when it comes to Early Years services. Moreover, it confirms the importance of letting Gypsies and Travellers speak for themselves in the planning of welfare services, unimpeded by preconceived integrationist agendas. We would concur with Hester's general conclusion for the Children's Fund.

> It is therefore pivotal that if inclusionary strategies are to be followed, then these need to be sensitively devised in order to ensure that these strategies, however well meaning and well resourced, are not undermined by the spectre of assimilation and are thus rejected by the very people for whom they are intended to benefit. (Hester 2004, p.48)

Implications for Children's Centres

- The unreflective application of political mantras about multiculturalism and inclusiveness is unlikely to produce popular or adequate provision; more detailed exploration of specific cultural norms, and associated needs, are required to create provision that successfully reaches minority populations.

- A mainstream model of service delivery may be more popular amongst service providers than it is amongst service users. This poses the question about who the social inclusion agenda is designed for, and whose perspective should be prioritised.

- There is greater need for on-site provision for Gypsy and Traveller communities, at least when it comes to Early Years services. Moreover, Gypsies and Travellers should be enabled to speak for themselves in the planning of welfare services.

References

Acton, T. (1974) *Gypsies, Politics and Social Change.* London: Routledge and Kegan Paul.

Adams, B., Okely, J., Morgan, D. and Smith, D. (1975) *Gypsies and Government Policy in England.* London: Heineman.

Department for Education and Skills (2005) *Ethnicity and Education: the Evidence on Minority Ethnic Pupils.* London: DfES.

Dwivedi, K. (2002) *Meeting the Needs of Ethnic Minority Children Including Refugee, Black and Mixed Parentage Children.* London: Jessica Kingsley Publishers.

Fisher, I. (2004) *Deprivation and Discrimination Faced by Traveller Children – Implications for Social Policy and Social Work.* Norwich: University of East Anglia.

Greenfields, M. (2006) 'Family, community and identity.' In C. Clark and M. Greenfields (2006), *Here to Stay: the Gypsies and Travellers of Britain.* Hatfield: University of Hertfordshire Press.

Hawes, D. and Perez, B. (1996) *The Gypsy and the State: The Ethnic Cleansing of British Society* (2nd edition) Bristol: Policy Press.

Hester, R. (2004) *Services Provided to Gypsy Traveller Children: a Review of the Current Literature for the National Evaluation of the Children's Fund.* Birmingham, NECF. www.ne-cf.org.uk/core_files/lit%20review%20GT%20final%20final30NOVEMBER.doc, accessed on 13 September 2006.

Home Office (2005) *Improving Opportunity, Strengthening Society: The Government's Strategy to Increase Race Equality and Community Cohesion.* London: Home Office.

Kelly, R. (2006) Speech by Ruth Kelly MP at the launch of the new Commission on Integration and Cohesion on 24 August 2006. www.communities.gov.uk/speeches/corporate/commision-integration-cohesion, accessed on 13 September 2006.

Levinson, M and Sparkes, A. (2003) 'Gypsy masculinities and the home–school interface: exploring contradictions and tensions.' *British Journal of Sociology of Education 24*, 5, 587–603.

Mason, P., Plumridge, G., Barnes, M., Beirens, H. and Broughton, K. (2006) *Preventative Services for Gypsy/Traveller Children.* Birmingham: NECF. Available atwww.ne-cf.org.uk/care_files/RR781.pdf, accessed on 13 September 2006.

McCarthy, P. (1994) 'The sub-culture of poverty reconsidered.' In M. McCann, O. Síocháin and J. Ruane (eds) *Irish Travellers: Culture and Ethnicity.* Belfast: Institute of Irish Studies.

Okely, J. (1983) *Changing Cultures: The Traveller Gypsies.* Cambridge: Cambridge University Press.

OFSTED (1996) *The Education of Travelling Children: a Survey of Educational Provision for Travelling Children.* London: OFSTED.

O'Hanlon, C. and Holmes, P. (2004) *The Education of Gypsy and Traveller Children: Towards Inclusion and Achievement.* Stoke: Trentham Books.

Sure Start Unit (2005) *The Origins of the Sure Start Programme.* www.surestart.gov.uk/surestartservices/settings/surestartlocalprogrammes/history/, accessed on 9 November 2007.

Worrall, D. (1979) *Gypsy Education: A Study of Provision in England and Wales.* Walsall: Council for Community Relations.

Chapter 26

Changing Conceptions
of Community

Max Hope and Paul Leighton

This chapter examines the changing conceptions of community that under-pinned Sure Start over the life of the programme and illustrates these using evaluation data from a number of schemes in the East Midlands.

It suggests that in its early days Sure Start was underpinned by a 'bounded' notion of community that stressed the desirability of homogeneous, cohesive, place-based communities, and which prioritised local participation in the management and delivery of Sure Start services. The chapter then tracks the emergence of a second, more 'porous', notion of community within New Labour thinking – one which stresses more strongly the significance of economic participation (especially through employment). We suggest that it is this second version of community that underpinned Sure Start from at least 2002 onwards and that led ultimately to the policy being dismantled. We conclude by suggesting that the transition to Children's Centres should be understood as the culmination of these developments.

To explore these issues the chapter draws upon a number of Sure Start Local Programme evaluations with which the authors have been directly or indirectly involved. Whilst these evaluations have necessarily been broad in substantive focus (for example, see Avis and Leighton 2003), have developed concerns for both processes and outcomes, and have most often been domi-nated by concerns for appropriate and effective service delivery, they do offer the potential to step back and reflect more broadly upon the local experience of Sure Start. This chapter draws upon a sample of semistructured interviews (approximately 30) carried out in five local Sure Start programmes between 2002 and 2007; these interviews were broadly focused upon organisational and management issues. The interviews were revisited utilising thematic analysis, with a particular concern for the concepts of *social exclusion, social cohesion, social capital* and *community*.

New Labour, the 'New Localism' and Community

'Community' both as a goal and as a mechanism for delivery has had a long history within social policy (Imrie and Raco 2003, p.4), and under New Labour and Third Way thinking it has taken on renewed significance.

Third Way thinking seeks to find a midpoint between the emphasis on individual responsibility found within Neo-Liberal arguments and the notion that The State should be a major provider of welfare provision, often emphasised within more left-leaning accounts. Within this thinking, it is 'community' that is the midpoint between the individual and The State – it is through 'the mobilisation of active communities' that social problems are addressed. This 'responsibilisation of community' has been characterised as a 'New Localism' and is a key feature of a wide range of developments within social policy under New Labour (Raco 2003).

Yet definitions of community and their rights and responsibilities are rarely static and uncontested. At times a 'place-based' definition has been called upon.

> Communities are often understood to exist in particular places and the aim of policy is to help them to help themselves. (Raco 2003, p.236)

In these terms the ideal community is characterised by a homogeneity of interests and clear geographic boundaries. Such communities are expected to help themselves by being actively represented in the local management of social policy initiatives such as Sure Start.

A new way of thinking about community participation in social policy, however, can also be found (Raco 2003). This stresses non-place-based communities and 'communities of interest' rather than geographically bounded notions of attachment and connection. These more 'porous' versions of community acknowledge how in a global economy people are part of social and economic worlds that transcend the boundaries of the particular locality within which they happen to be located. In these circumstances people often have weak ties with their immediate neighbours and stronger ties with members of wider geographically dispersed communities of interest (i.e. through work, through hobbies and past-times, and facilitated by improved communication and transport links). Evidence of this kind of understanding can be found in the government's Community Strategies initiative launched in 2000.

> Individuals belong simultaneously to a number of communities of interest, of both place and interest, and will identify with different communities according to their circumstances and the issues under discussion. Community Strategies should reflect this complexity and...accommodate it by putting in place a variety of routes into participation. (Department of Environment, Transport and Regions 2001, cited in Raco 2003, p. 239)

Cameron (2005) suggests that in this version of community people are responsible for their participation in the wider economic community rather than the self-management of the local community.

In this chapter we argue that in its early stages Sure Start tended to work with geographically 'bounded' notions of community of the sort described above. In its later manifestations, however, we suggest that it has increasingly drawn upon more 'porous' versions of community, and that this is at times the source of some tension and difficulties for managers and service users.

Sure Start and bounded communities

Sure Start has its origins in a Comprehensive Spending Review carried out by the new Labour government in 1998 where it was conceived as a family support programme for parents in deprived areas (Glass 1999). A separate Sure Start Unit was created and managed jointly by the Department of Health and the Department for Education and Employment (now the Department for Children, Schools and Families (DCSF)). Communities were selected to develop Sure Start Local Programmes according to deprivation levels, and local management boards were set up that brought together key local stakeholders (local authorities, education authorities, health boards, etc.) and representatives of the community to manage these schemes. At this initial stage Sure Start Programmes had four objectives: improving social and emotional development, improving health, improving children's ability to learn, and strengthening families and communities. The latter was to be achieved by involving families in creating and managing Sure Start Local Programmes, and by developing the community's capacity independently to sustain social and healthcare activities and initiatives post-Sure Start funding. To these ends all Sure Start programmes had to have parent representatives on their local management board.

In geographically targeting resources, in managing services in an integrated manner (using local stakeholders and community members), and in looking to strengthen community capacity and social cohesion, it is clear that at these early stages Sure Start drew heavily upon place-based definitions of community. As the Sure Start guidance indicated:

> Sure Start is rooted in particular places, in coherent neighbourhoods, the boundaries of which are clearly defined (and which) make sense to local people. (Department for Education and Skills 2002)

This emphasis on shared locality and on developing participation and social cohesion within these boundaries was born out by those working within Sure Start settings.

> We have this huge amount of vulnerable people *in our community*...a lot of poverty. What you would want them to do is to have a piece of the pie and try and convince them that it is worth doing. (Christine, Sure Start Manager)

> Sure Start [is] run in partnership with parents. They...can affect what goes on. It is a place where you can get support for any number of issues. (Karen, Sure Start staff member)

Perhaps more significantly it was validated by those who accessed Sure Start services and provision (Glass 2005).

> It's the first time I felt like that 'like professionals want your opinion'. Professionals really care about what you think. It's like this morning I had to miss a group but [the person running the group] rang and told me what went on...they are very keen on what we want. (Joanne, Sure Start parent)

For some, an important aspect of this process was the development of a stronger sense of local attachment and local friendships – the development of a sense of local community.

> [Before Sure Start] I just felt that I was a put-upon parent. *Now I'm a valued member of the community...* I think I was just very kind of closed, closed and reclusive, like just with my family. Y'know I was stuck in the house with the kids, it was too much time just with the kids... I'm more confident and outgoing now. I know how to conduct myself properly with other people. *I feel that I am a valued member of the community.* (Tony, Sure Start parent)

> Sure Start's role *is to bring communities together* and to encourage them to get on with each other and perhaps become more friendlier, more sharing, go to groups, not our groups but *just build a whole community together.* (Sharon, Sure Start staff member)

Comments like these support the view that throughout the life of the programme Sure Start drew heavily upon geographically bounded notions of community, notions of community which stressed social homogeneity, shared circumstances and the benefits of working together to address social and economic problems. We would argue, however, that as Sure Start developed, this overriding sense of *community development* and *community cohesion* came to be replaced by a more open and porous sense of community and social connectivity.

Communities, globalisation and 'the logic of no alternative'

Initiatives such as Sure Start cannot be understood independently of the broader social and political context within which they are constructed. In the case of Sure Start it lies in an agenda for the eradication of childhood poverty (Walker 1999, esp. chapter by Tony Blair; for more on this see Leighton and Hope 2007) but also in the *rapidly developing* New Labour, Third Way approach to social policy: '[the early years of the Labour government] focused on undoing the damage visited on the UK by 13 years of Conservatism...then the focus has shifted rapidly ever since' (Cameron 2005). This evolving focus rests in the inevitability of Neo-Liberal globalisation and the need for individuals to assume greater responsibility so that they are able to participate in an increasingly competitive economic environment, over which national governments have limited control. This is 'the logic of no alternative' as 'Labour's leaders appropriate...the image of a structurally weakened state necessarily ceding economic power to market imperatives' (Watson and Hay 2003, p.301).

This shift in focus has brought with it an emphasis on a new 'porous' sense of community. To be successful in the global economy, community boundaries need to become more open, and individuals better able to access broader, looser networks of social and economic opportunity.

> More and more people are suggesting that the supposed tight knit communities of the past are not what is needed in society today. Successful communities are characterised as much by weak as strong ties, both within the neighbourhood and across their boundaries. People need many overlapping networks which give them choice beyond their locality. (Taylor 2004)

These are communities of economic interest (and economic opportunity) which *span holes in the social and economic structure* rather than being confined by geographic boundaries and social similarity. Policies are required which link disadvantaged communities to the wider society, rather introspectively turning them in on themselves (for a broad review of these issues see Phillipson, Allan and Morgan 2004). Thus community participation has become redefined as participation in the wider economy, rather than the local self-management, which was a feature of earlier place-bound definitions.

A corresponding shift in the way that social exclusion is understood one which stresses behavioural explanations that emphasise personal failing (and in particular economic inactivity) – is also evident in evolving New Labour policy (Cameron 2005; Deacon 2003). Social exclusion, and by association childhood poverty, rest less in the inequities of the social and economic structures but are the result of individual behaviour and a failure to take, or even seek, avenues of economic opportunity.

> The poor and marginal are presented less as victims of multiple chronic, socioeconomic processes, and more as the 'inactive', the 'unviable', the uncompetitive: those who do not...play by the rules. (Cameron 2005, p.198)

This section of the chapter has suggested a number of changes to the way in which community and social exclusion have been conceptualised within evolving New Labour social policy. The next section considers the way in which these have been reflected in changes to the organisation and delivery of Sure Start.

Sure Start and porous communities

This shift to a porous definition of community within Sure Start (and associated concerns for economic activity) became manifest in two interconnected ways:

the 'mainstreaming' of Sure Start services since 2002, and the increased importance given to childcare and the employability agenda over the same period.

Hastings (2003) in her account of New Labour's neighbourhood renewal policy suggests that the mainstreaming of services is indicative of a shift in thinking from *inward-looking* area-based policies to a more *outward-looking*, strategic approach 'that emphasises the role of mainstream government and public sector activity in determining the trajectory of neighbourhoods' (2003, p.85). Stronger involvement from local authorities, as they assume responsibility for new multi-level regional regeneration partnerships, marks a clear and direct scaling up of the level at which solutions to neighbourhood problems are perceived to lie. Solutions are no longer seen to lie with neighbourhoods (within communities) but are seen to require action at a regional, or at least local authority, level. Thus the 'mainstreaming of services' might be interpreted as a response to the increasingly global and complex nature of the problems facing neighbourhoods, and indicative of New Labour's increasing preference for porous over bounded definitions of community, i.e. linking neighbourhoods regionally, rather than isolating them locally.

Since at least 2002 there has been a similar drift away from the notion of Sure Start as locally managed stand-alone programmes as they have increasingly been incorporated into mainstream services, with more direct and identifiable links to other statutory service agencies. This process began with a comprehensive spending review in 2002 when Sure Start became the joint responsibility of the then Department of Education and Skills (now the Department of Children, Schools and Families) and the Department of Work and Pensions. This signalled the end of the role of the Department of Health and the beginnings of the incorporation of Sure Start within the government's childcare strategy. Naomi Eisenstadt (2006), the government's Chief Adviser on Children and Young People's Services up to the end of 2006, characterised this as the *mainstreaming* of Sure Start as 'a move from alleviating poverty to eliminating poverty…[through] a strong employment and childcare agenda'. Sure Start programmes were to have a new role in providing childcare provision which would allow parents to juggle work and family responsibilities, thus tackling social exclusion through employment.

The mainstreaming of Sure Start and the development of this childcare agenda have developed hand in hand throughout this period. *Every Child Matters* (Department for Education and Skills 2003) signalled a desire that all organisations providing services for children should do so in an integrated (*mainstreamed*) fashion, rather than in isolation from each other. A Ten-Year Strategy for Childcare (HM Treasury 2004) has made a commitment to high quality childcare for children between the ages of 3 and 14. Targets focused upon the child's social, emotional and communication skills and upon the availability and take-up of childcare suggest a more restricted and focused agenda (*Times Educational Supplement* 15 April 2005).

The twin processes of mainstreaming Sure Start provision and developing a childcare/employability agenda has meant that Sure Start has travelled a long way from the notion of self-contained, locally managed programmes that it started with. Instead, a stronger emphasis upon employability, and an associated concern for the provision of childcare to facilitate this, point to a very different type of initiative. For Norman Glass, one of the original architects of the Sure Start agenda, this has meant that Sure Start has been 'abolished in all but name' (*The Times* 8 March 2005). Elsewhere he has succinctly summarised the magnitude of the changes that the programme has experienced.

> What started off as a family support programme for parents in deprived areas has become a programme in which the important thing is to get people back into work, with a focus on childcare services and employability. (*Times Educational Supplement* 15 April 2005).

By 2005 a stronger concern for employability and childcare provision meant that concerns for geographically bounded and socially integrated communities had been replaced by a more evident focus upon the individual, and upon liberating the individual (both adult and child) from their local circumstances. This transition, and the contradictions and tensions that it has created, have not been lost on those who work within, alongside or simply access Sure Start Local Programmes.

First of all, in relation to mainstreaming, the tension between embedded local 'Sure Start ways of working' and the requirements and protocols of other service providers suggests a far from seamless transition. At the simplest level responsibilities might differ: 'I think the focus of Sure Start has been just 0–4 and young families, whereas we have a much broader remit' (Jane, family/community worker). However, different approaches and different ways of working can be more fundamental.

> For example child protection documentation is "you will do this, bang, bang, bang" and it is not deviated from. Whereas Sure Start it is like "we don't need to document this, we are not actively [formally] involved"…it is not because people are being difficult, but they haven't been aware of what is expected here. (Karl, social services)

Conflicts between Sure Start's previous broader agenda and its more restricted (employment-focused) form have also been an area where Sure Start staff have recognised some contradiction.

> I struggle with the agenda of getting people back into work, and poverty will be solved by people working, but that depends on what job they are doing, if they are packing shelves at a supermarket I don't think that is a valuable job, I don't think that that helps people's health. (Vicky, Sure Start Local Programme health lead)

A similar tension was identified in the National Evaluation of Sure Start report on employability.

> [Some Sure Start programmes]…perceive a tension between encouraging parents to go out to work and supporting the belief of many parents that part of being a good parent is to be at home with children when they are young. (Meadows and Garbers 2004)

Consequently the challenge of actively moving the agenda on has not been without its difficulties.

> One thing that they lack is focusing upon that increasing employability objective…the events that they run aren't always vocational type courses, it is often things that people like to do, which you might class as community involvement, but you can only go so far with that. There has to be a stage when you say "Right you've done flower arranging, can we move you onto looking at work, or maybe an IT course?" It is difficult, of course, because parents are there voluntarily, they will attend what they want to attend. [This programme has been responsive to what people want], they do a lot of work around asking what parents want, so if they are not saying about looking for work then what can we do? (Julie, Job Centre Plus)

This section has charted how broader changes in the priorities and focus of social policy have been manifest in the life of Sure Start, and have been the site of tension and difficulty.

Conclusion: the transition to Children's Centres

The purpose of this chapter has been to contextualise Sure Start and to demonstrate how an evolving policy agenda has influenced its development and has at times been the source of some uncertainty and difficulties for those involved in local programmes.

We started by recognising the importance of ideas of community to contemporary social policy and suggested that Sure Start has its origins in a very different conception of community to that which now underpins government policy on social exclusion and child poverty. Sure Start was conceived as a series of local programmes rooted in distinctive, geographically bounded communities; it was about rebuilding communities and enabling local people to take control of the services which affected their lives. More latterly concerns for Neo-Liberalism and economic competitiveness have challenged this agenda, and have brought to the fore stronger concerns for economic activity and the significance of employment. The community of this way of thinking is more porous and geographically wide-reaching; it is simply the network of connections and interactions that enables individuals to participate in the broader economic sphere. For Sure Start this has meant a stronger concern for the provision of childcare, and also for the mainstreaming of services under local authority direction.

We close this chapter by commenting upon how the emergence of Children's Centres consolidates these processes and can be seen as a culmination of these trends. 2006/2007 has seen the end of Sure Start Local Programmes as they have been incorporated into a broader world of local authority-led, multi-agency working – i.e. Children's Centres. Similar to Sure Start Local Programmes, Children's Centres are to act as a hub for fully integrated child and family services, incorporating health, education and family support. However, rather than being managed at the neighbourhood level, with independent budgets, they are to be incorporated into a more dispersed, but inter-connected, network of local authority-managed provision. The distinctiveness, and local responsiveness, of Sure Start Local Programmes (i.e. their concern for the *local community*) are potentially being replaced by concerns for universal services and service delivery targets (i.e. their very own *community of shared interests*). Furthermore, more restricted funding and a stronger focus upon childcare (to enable parents back into work) and upon educational outcomes for both parents and children (to create better qualified workers) suggests an agenda where former concerns for community development and community cohesion are less significant than emergent concerns for individual economic activity.

Describing the wider policy context, as we have here, helps us to understand why Sure Start was eventually dismantled and replaced by Children's Centres – not because Sure Start had been successful, nor because it had failed but because the broader agenda had shifted. Awareness of this broader, and perhaps still shifting, policy backdrop offers us possibly a more effective map upon which to chart the development and success of the Children's Centres agenda as it grows.

Implications for Children's Centres

- The transition from Sure Start Local Programme provision to Children's Centre provision should be considered neither as a mark of success nor of failure but is rather symptomatic of broader trends in changing governmental, social policy agenda.

- Sure Start Local Programmes and Children's Centres cannot be divorced from broader patterns and trends in social and healthcare policy provision. Therefore, to understand these initiatives fully we have to engage with notions such as *community, social exclusion, social cohesion*, etc. which are influential in shaping the broader policy arena.

- A focus upon childcare, education and employability, as manifest in the Children's Centre agenda, should not be accepted uncritically; they are just one set of solutions, to one possible way of conceptualising the issues at stake.

References

Avis, M. and Leighton, P. (2003) *Local Evaluation of Sure Start St Ann's – first report.* www.ness.bbk.ac.uk/documents/annualreports/1278.pdf, accessed on 16 April 2007.

Cameron, A. (2005) 'Geographies of welfare and exclusion: initial report', *Progress in Human Geography 29,* 2, 194–203.

Deacon, A. (2003) 'Levelling the playing field, activating the players: New Labour and the cycle of disadvantage.' *Policy and Politics 31,* 2, 123–137.

Department for Education and Skills (2002) *Sure Start, A Guide for Sixth Wave Programmes.* Nottingham: DfES Publications.

Department for Education and Skills (2003) *Every Child Matters* Cm 5860. London: The Stationery Office.

Eisenstadt, N. (2006) 'What we know from the National Evaluation of Sure Start.' Conference presentation at *Learning from Sure Start. National Conference on Local Evaluations* 14–15 June, Nottingham.

Glass, N. (1999) 'Sure Start: the development of an early intervention programme for young children in the United Kingdom.' *Children and Society 13,* 257–264.

Glass, N. (2005) 'Surely Some Mistake', *Society Guardian,* 5 January.

Hastings, A. (2003) 'Strategic, multi-level neighbourhood regeneration: an outward-looking approach at last?' In R. Imrie and M. Raco *Urban Renaissance: New Labour, Community and Urban Policy.* Bristol: Policy Press.

HM Treasury (2004) *Choice for Parents, the Best Start for Children: A Ten-year Strategy for Childcare.* London: HM Treasury.

Imrie, R. and Raco, M. (2003) *Urban Renaissance: New Labour, Community and Urban Policy.* Bristol: Policy Press.

Meadows, P. and Garbers, C. (2004) *National Evaluation Report 6 – Improving the Employability of Parents in Sure Start Local Programmes.* Nottingham: DfES Publications.

Phillipson, C., Allan, G. and Morgan, D. (2004) *Social Networks and Social Exclusion – Sociological and Policy Perspectives.* Aldershot: Ashgate.

Raco, M. (2003) 'New Labour, community and the future of Britain's urban renaissance.' In R. Imrie and M. Raco *Urban Renaissance: New Labour, Community and Urban Policy.* Bristol: Policy Press.

Taylor, M. (2004) 'Community issues and social networks.' In C. Phillipson, G. Allan and D. Morgan *Social Networks and Social Exclusion – Sociological and Policy Perspectives.* Aldershot: Ashgate.

Times Educational Supplement (2005) 'Limited evidence for Sure Start's progress. *Times Education Supplement,* 15 April 2005.

The Times (2005) 'Sure Start's end is in sight.' *The Times,* 8 March 2005. www.timesonline.co.uk/tol/life_and_style/career_and_jobs/public_sector/article420794.ece, accessed on 12 November 2007.

Walker, R. (1999) *Ending Child Poverty: Popular Welfare for the 21st Century?* Bristol: Policy Press.

Watson, M. and Hay, C. (2003) 'The discourse of globalisation and the logic of no alternative: rendering the contingent necessary in the political economy of New Labour. *Policy and Politics 31,* 3, 289–305.

Conclusion: Lessons from Sure Start Local Programmes

Justine Schneider, Mark Avis and Paul Leighton

The Sure Start initiative, from 1999 to 2004, can be seen as a landmark experiment in Early Years services. Many of its lessons have already been assimilated into practice and other longer-term results remain to be analysed. In this book we offer a collection of themed chapters, each of which encapsulates some of the experience of Sure Start Local Programmes (SSLPs). We hope that, together, they will provide reference points for Children's Centres and at the same time document the Sure Start experience. In order to make the lessons from Sure Start transferable to other initiatives, many of the authors present their findings from an explicit theoretical perspective. This provides a framework for understanding and analysis which may be applied to other settings. A shared perspective enables comparisons to be made and general inferences to be drawn. With this, the learning derived from Children's Centres can build upon the Sure Start experience to increase our knowledge about how to work more effectively with children and families.

The *Ten Year Strategy for Childcare* (HM Treasury 2004) brought a policy shift, from the targeting of disadvantaged communities and families that was characteristic of the original Sure Start, to a promise of universal provision with a 'Sure Start Children's Centre' in every community by 2010. Children's Centres in disadvantaged areas have additional responsibilities, outlined in Box 1, which is what is meant by 'universalism with a targeted approach' (the then Minister for Children, Margaret Hodge, at the 2003 Sure Start conference).

Besides this modified universalism, a second important difference is that Children's Centres do not necessarily share the emphasis placed by Sure Start on parental involvement and community development, discussed throughout this book. We would argue that this poses a danger of losing sight of the learning from Sure Start in relation to strengthening families and communities. If that happens, these insights may have to be rediscovered by Children's Centres through trial and error at a later stage. The sections on working in partnership with parents and on developing communities are offered here, despite the fact that they are not an explicit priority of Children's Centres, in an effort to document some of the progress made by SSLPs.

For instance, the Sure Start experience demonstrates that in many cases working through parents as peer supporters and educators is more acceptable and therefore likely to be more effective than a top-down approach by professionals. This is illustrated here in the chapters by Griffin and Carpenter (11),

---

Box 1 Responsibilities of Sure Start Children's Centres in the most disadvantaged areas

Sure Start Children's Centres in the most disadvantaged areas will offer the following services:

- good quality early learning combined with full day care provision for children (minimum ten hours a day, five days a week, 48 weeks a year)
- good quality teacher input to lead the development of learning within the centre
- child and family health services, including ante-natal services
- parental outreach
- family support services
- a base for a childminder network
- support for children and parents with special needs, and
- effective links with Jobcentre Plus to support parents/carers who wish to consider training or employment.

In more advantaged areas, although local authorities will have flexibility in which services they provide to meet local need, all Sure Start Children's Centres will have to provide a minimum range of services including:

- appropriate support and outreach services to parents/carers and children who have been identified as in need of them
- information and advice to parents/carers on a range of subjects, including: local childcare, looking after babies and young children, local Early Years provision (childcare and early learning) education services for three and four-year-olds
- support to childminders
- drop-in sessions and other activities for children and carers at the centre
- links to Jobcentre Plus services.

Potter (4), Perry (3), Thurston (18), Graham (10) and Wigfall *et al.* (9). These lessons imply that Children's Centres might consider working with and through parents and should bear in mind the importance of not seeming to patronise them.

Second, local communities or cultures have clearly affected the implementation of Sure Start and the means to successful working which have been identified. Hope and Leighton (Chapter 26) discuss the meaning of community and how this has evolved. Despite a reduced emphasis on community as such, there are empirical lessons to be drawn from Sure Start. For example, many SSLPs have shown that activities designed to appeal to broad groups of people – adult learning, outings, holiday clubs, fetes and sports events – can help to engage families who would avoid formal services. Cullen and Lindsay (Chapter 15), Featherstone, Manby and Nicholls (20), Carman *et al.* (5) and McKenna (21) all argue that it is crucial to meet people on their own terms, to be non-judgemental and to take services to families. Sure Start has struggled to gear services to needs through the close involvement of parents on SSLP Management Boards, with variable success. Hamm's chapter (24) analyses some of the problems, and the dynamics of professionals working alongside parents are discussed by Cullen and Lindsay. All of these chapters raise issues for Children's Centres: how to embed services in relation to the local population, how to present them to maximise access, and how to ensure that they are appropriate.

Of course, Children's Centres and their predecessor SSLPs have many objectives in common: health promotion, family support, and parental employment, for example, and these themes constitute a substantial part of this book. These chapters will inevitably present questions that have already posed challenges to Sure Start: how to involve men, how best to work with hard-to-reach families, how to work in partnership with mainstream providers, what is multidisciplinary working and how to monitor outputs and outcomes. Evaluation easily slips down a manager's list of things to do. Barton, Jesson and Horton draw attention to some lessons from Sure Start about monitoring and measurement (Chapter 22).

Experience from SSLPs points to the value of specialist practitioners offering training to Children's Centre staff. This has been shown to be effective in relation to problems which are easier to resolve through early recognition, and in relation to topics that are particularly sensitive. Potter and Hodgson (Chapter 6) demonstrate the potential of training by specialist speech and language therapists to provide communication enriched environments for pre-school children. Hall and Finnigan (7) illustrate how training in maternal mental health issues can support early recognition and response to signs of distress.

Some of the ingenuity and creativity of SSLPs in engaging families is illustrated in Pearson and Martin's chapter (16). This also presents one of the rare Sure Start forays into the domain of adult education, which has moved centre stage in the Ten Year Strategy for Childcare. Featherstone, Manby and Nicholls, McKenna, and Thurston focus on access to services, while Bowpitt and Chaudhary (Chapter 25) address the issues from the perspective of multiculturalism. Although they write about Travellers, their approach may be applied to any distinctive group. Many of the chapters in this book stress the importance of outreach in delivering the benefits of innovative services, ensuring that people are aware of services, understand them and feel confident in accessing them. We believe that it is essential that Children's Centres can assimilate the learning that SSLPs have generated about successful outreach.

Edgley's analysis of the interface between SSLPs and mainstream services (Chapter 12) has direct application to Children's Centres, while Griffin and Carpenter highlight some of the processes which can facilitate joint working. The relationships between professionals working in different agencies may need as much attention as the relationships between parents and Children's Centres. Moreover, the ability to mobilise the resources of partner agencies will be vital to Children Centres' attainment of their goals.

One general conclusion is to be drawn from the evidence collected in this book. There is a need to develop a theoretical understanding of the practical innovations that Sure Start has promoted. This relates both to the values which are embodied in day-to-day practice and to the theories of change espoused by services. Examples of differing value systems are shown in the debates around universalism versus targeting (e.g. Edgley), around user involvement versus professional leadership (e.g. Cullen and Lindsay) and around what we mean by community (Hope and Leighton (Chapter 26); Hamm (24); Bowpitt and Chaudhary (25)). Second, an understanding of how interventions are believed to achieve a programme's goals has seldom been articulated in SSLPs. Barton *et al.* point out that evaluation of such programmes demands a shared, robust theory of how such services are thought to make a difference to families.

Future services for children might benefit not only from reflecting on the philosophy which underpins what they do, but also from developing a statement of principles which guide their work. An explicit statement of values of this kind can help services to respond to new incentives and to navigate though changing conditions. Those people responsible for implementing services might also consider *how* what they do makes a difference to children and families; what mechanisms bring about the changes to which they aspire. An explicit, evidence-based theory of change could help them to prioritise objectives and to engage mainstream services. Ultimately, a clear understanding of what ought to be happening and how it is meant to be brought about will make it possible for services to evaluate and improve their effectiveness.

Reference

HM Treasury (2004) *Choice for Parent, the Best Start for Children: a Ten Year Strategy for Childcare.* Norwich: HMSO.

Contributors

Mark Avis is currently Professor of Social Contexts of Health at the School of Nursing at the University of Nottingham. His research career has focussed on the use of qualitative research techniques to explore people's experiences of health and social care. He has led a number of local evaluations of Sure Start programmes in the East Midlands.

Paul Leighton is a research fellow based in the Trent RDSU at the University of Nottingham. He is a sociologist who has an interest in the application of concepts such as social exclusion and social capital to health and social care research and service delivery. Between 2002–2007 he was based at the School of Nursing at the University of Nottingham where he was involved in a number of Sure Start Local Programme evaluations.

Justine Schneider is Professor of Mental Health and Social Care in the School of Sociology and Social Policy, University of Nottingham, and Nottinghamshire Healthcare NHS Trust. From 2000–2005 she was a member of the Durham University Sure Start evaluation team, working particularly on the costs and outcomes of SSLPs in Darlington and County Durham.

Anne Barton is currently Head of Social Research and Corporate Performance at M•E•L Research. Anne has managed the majority of M•E•L's Sure Start and Children's Centre portfolio since the late 1990s. In addition to over 25 consultations and evaluations on behalf of Sure Start Local Programmes and Children's Centres, Anne manages research, consultation and evaluation projects for a wide range of other public service clients.

Janet Boddy *see* Valerie Wigfall

Graham Bowpitt is Senior Lecturer in Social Policy at Nottingham Trent University. He has managed the local evaluation of five local Sure Start programmes from the beginning of 2003 to late 2007.

Julie Carman is the manager of the Accident Prevention Team for East Lancashire Primary Care Trust. Her current responsibilities include managing the Accident Prevention Team and developing and delivering initiatives to reduce and prevent accidental injury. The team provides a Home Safety Equipment Scheme to over 1000 families each year and outreach training and advice on accident prevention across the area using a multi-agency approach.

John Carpenter is Professor of Social Work and Applied Social Science, University of Bristol. He was previously Professor and Director of the Centre for Applied Social and Community Studies, Durham University and led the family support and Sure Start research programme from 2000 until 2005.

Sarah Chaudhary is a research associate at the University of Nottingham. She worked as an evaluator at four Nottinghamshire Sure Start programmes between 2002 and 2007.

Brian Crosbie is research associate in the School of Nursing, University of Nottingham. He has worked on a number of Sure Start local evaluation projects and was previously an evaluation officer for a Sure Start Local Programme in Derby. He is currently working with the Sue Ryder Centre for Palliative Care and End of Life Studies.

Mairi Ann Cullen is a senior research fellow in the Centre for Educational Development, Appraisal and Research (CEDAR) at the University of Warwick. Under the direction of Professor Geoff Lindsay, she conducted the 2004 local evaluation of Sure Start Chelmsley Wood.

Alison Edgley is a social science lecturer in the School of Nursing at the University of Nottingham. She has evaluated a number of Sure Start services from the perspective of statutory service providers in the Nottinghamshire area.

Brid Featherstone is Professor of Social Work and Social Policy at the University of Bradford. She has been involved in evaluating Sure Start Bramley for the last six years and has completed a range of other evaluations in the areas of family support and assessment.

Marjorie Finnigan is a mental health worker at Sure Start Salford. She works with clinical psychologists and a counsellor as part of The Perinatal Mental Health Project in order to provide a service to women experiencing perinatal depression.

Ellis Friedman is Director of Public Health, East Lancashire Primary Care Trust and North West Regional Director of Breast Screening Quality Assurance. His major interests are in screening, coronary heart disease and cancer. He qualified in medicine at Manchester University in 1977 and is a Fellow of the Faculty of Public Health.

Alissa Goodman is a deputy director of the Institute for Fiscal Studies and Director of the Education, Employment and Evaluation research sector. **Barbara Sianesi** is a Senior Research Economist in the Education, Employment and Evaluation research sector. Though not directly involved in the evaluation of the Sure Start intervention, they have worked extensively on assessing the longer-term impacts of early education on the cognitive, social, educational and labour market attainment of a cohort of British children born in 1958.

Pamela Graham is currently a principal lecturer and the director for the Children's Agenda in the School of Health, Community and Education Studies at Northumbria University. Having previously worked in and managed multi-agency family support services, Pamela's vested interest in the Sure Start philosophy led to her involvement in the evaluation of a number of local programmes.

Michaela Griffin works on the Master of Social Work Programme at Durham University and for the Commission for Social Care Inspection. As a senior research associate in the Durham University Centre for Applied Social Research, she worked on evaluations of various children's services and partnership initiatives, including an evaluation of the impact of Sure Start on referrals to social services, a project commissioned by the DfES.

Pauline Hall is a clinical psychologist working in the NHS and Sure Start in Salford, Greater Manchester. Her clinical work includes the assessment and delivery of psychological interventions for antenatal and postnatal women. Her work also includes consultation, teaching, research and supervision in relation to maternal mental health issues.

Tricia Hamm is completing her PhD which has focussed on the assumptions about human agency within Sure Start and Third Way policy discourses. She is a researcher with several years' experience of researching issues around 'inclusion' and inequalities, and has recently completed a study about Sure Start Plus services for pregnant teenagers and teenage parents.

Kate Hardman is a senior research officer in the East Lancashire Public Health Resource and Intelligence Centre. Prior to this she worked as a Research and Information Officer for the British Fluoridation Society. She has a particular interest in health inequalities.

Sharon Hodgson is Principal Speech and Language Therapist for County Durham Primary Care Trust. She has been working with a Sure Start Local Programme for the last five years on speech and language issues.

Max Hope is Deputy Head of the Department of Geography and Development Studies at the University of Chester. He is researching geographical aspects of social exclusion, including the role of local communities in service management and delivery.

Matthew Horton is Performance Management and Evaluation Officer for the Early Years and Childcare Service at Stoke-on-Trent City Council.

Jill Jesson is currently a lecturer in managing public health to undergraduates, and applied research to postgraduates, at Aston Business School, University of Aston. In her capacity as Principal Consultant in Health and Social Care to M•E•L Research, Jill has undertaken research and evaluation over 20 years in many community development and health-based projects.

David Lamb is Head of the East Lancashire Public Health Resource and Intelligence Centre. He has 16 years' experience of information management and public health data analysis. He has a special interest in child poverty issues and the effects on adult health of deprivation in childhood.

Geoff Lindsay is Director of the Centre for Educational Development, Appraisal and Research (CEDAR) at the University of Warwick where he is Professor of Educational Psychology and Special Education Needs.

Martin Manby is Director of Nationwide Children's Research Centre, Huddersfield, West Yorkshire.

Ann Martin *see* Mathew Pearson

Lynne McKenna is Principal Lecturer for the Wider Workforce in the School of Health, Community and Education Studies at Northumbria University. Prior to joining the University, she taught throughout the Early Years departments in schools in South Tyneside. She is currently researching the ways in which Early Years area-based interventions, such as Family Learning programmes, Sure Start and Education Action Zones, impact upon the communities they are designed for.

Susan McQuail *see* Valerie Wigfall

Nicky Nicholls has been working as a health visitor for 23 years. She was a member of the original development team for Sure Start Bramley and has been a member of the team for over six years. During this time she has worked very closely with the evaluation team.

Matthew Pearson and **Ann Martin** run Impact Research Solutions, an independent company specialising in research and evaluation work in the fields of social welfare and education.

Catherine Perry is Deputy Director of the Centre for Public Health Research and Postgraduate Programme Leader in Research Methods at the University of Chester. Her research work has included: the evaluation of various innovative nursing roles, evaluative work with local Healthy Living Centre initiatives, and evaluative work with Sure Start Local Programmes.

Carol Potter is Senior Lecturer at the Carnegie Faculty of Sport and Education, part of Leeds Metropolitan University. Carol trained as a nursery teacher before moving into the field of research where she has undertaken several research projects in the area of language and communication development. For six years she was a research fellow at Durham University, leading a county-wide longitudinal evaluation of a number of local Sure Start programmes.

Barbara Sianesi *see* Alissa Goodman

Miranda Thurston is Professor of Public Health and Director of the Centre for Public Health Research at the University of Chester. Miranda has a specific interest in evaluation methodology, developed through her involvement in a number of commissioned evaluation studies concerned with the implementation of national policy initiatives at a local level. This has involved designing evaluation strategies for Sure Start and Children's Fund local programmes, as well as for specific interventions such as exercise on prescription schemes.

Valerie Wigfall and **Janet Boddy** are research officers and **Susan McQuail** is a research associate at the Thomas Coram Research Unit, Institute of Education, University of London. Between them, they have completed many Sure Start Local Evaluations since the commencement of the programme in 1999.

Subject Index

Author Index